BUSINESS BUILDERS

IN COSMETICS

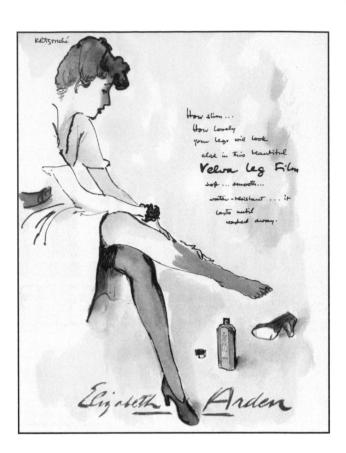

A 1943 Elizabeth Arden ad for Velva Leg Film. During World War II, stocking material was rationed, so women sometimes painted their legs instead of wearing hosiery.

BUSINESS BUILDERS

BUSINESS BUILDERS IN BROADCASTING
BUSINESS BUILDERS IN COMPUTERS
BUSINESS BUILDERS IN COSMETICS
BUSINESS BUILDERS IN FASHION
BUSINESS BUILDERS IN FAST FOOD
BUSINESS BUILDERS IN OIL
BUSINESS BUILDERS IN REAL ESTATE
BUSINESS BUILDERS IN SWEETS AND TREATS
BUSINESS BUILDERS IN TOYS AND GAMES

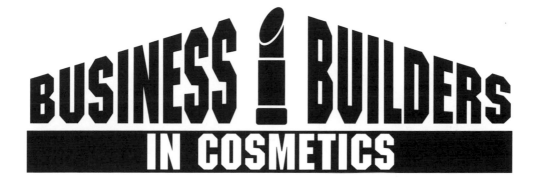

BUSINESS BUILDERS
IN COSMETICS

Jacqueline C. Kent

The Oliver Press, Inc.
Minneapolis

For Rachael, my sister, my protector, and my friend.

© 2004 by The Oliver Press, Inc.

The Oliver Press, Inc.
Charlotte Square
5707 West 36th Street
Minneapolis, MN 55416-2510

Library of Congress Cataloging-in-Publication Data

Kent, Jacqueline C.
    Business builders in cosmetics / Jacqueline C. Kent.
       p. cm. — (Business builders ; 7)
    Summary: Describes the history of cosmetics and profiles seven cosmetics entrepreneurs,
including Helen Rubinstein, Elizabeth Arden, and Max Factor.
    Includes bibliographical references and index.
    ISBN 1-881508-82-X
    1. Cosmetics industry—History—Juvenile literature. 2.
Businesspeople—Biography—Juvenile literature. [1. Cosmetics industry. 2.
Businesspeople.] I. Title. II. Series.

HD9970.5.C672K46 2004
338.7'6164672'0922—dc21

                                                                    2002041033
                                                              CIP
                                                              AC

ISBN 1-881508-82-X
Printed in the United States of America

10 09 08 07 06 05 04   8 7 6 5 4 3 2 1

CONTENTS

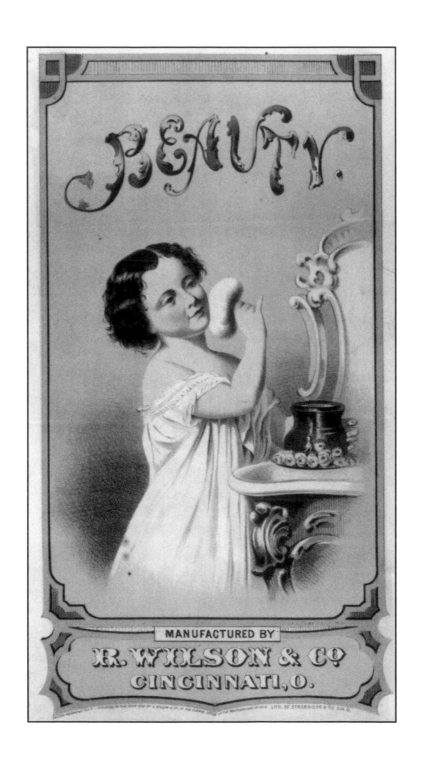

INTRODUCTION

COSMETICS: DEMEANING VERSUS EMPOWERING

From Queen Nefertiti of Egypt to Hollywood's Marilyn Monroe, women have used cosmetics to protect their skin and enhance or alter their appearances. The beauty secrets they freely shared with one another eventually evolved into an industry that today commands billions of dollars each year in the United States and Canada.

Throughout history, some people have believed that the use of cosmetics empowered women, while others condemned it for demeaning them. Cosmetics can mask or diminish imperfections and allow women to express themselves, feel more beautiful, and be self-confident. On the other hand, some people believe that cosmetic use places too much importance on a woman's physical appearance, and

Face powder is one of the oldest and most basic cosmetics. It was also one of the first "acceptable" beauty products in the modern era. This ad dates from 1869.

may make her feel inadequate by setting unattainable standards. Some women went to great lengths to hide the fact that they used cosmetics, while others proudly flaunted their use. For some, purchasing expensive brands allowed them the fantasy of being part of an exclusive level of society; others took advantage of the business opportunities offered by the cosmetics industry to actually enter into those elite levels of society. Whether perceived as good or bad, from the first time people added paint or color to their bodies, cosmetics have affected world cultures on numerous levels.

COSMETICS IN THE BEGINNING

Our early ancestors believed they could make themselves more terrifying and protect themselves from evil forces by drawing scary designs on their faces. Paint was also used to frighten human enemies. In Africa and South America, various tribes painted their bodies when they went hunting or on war expeditions. When Europeans first traveled to Africa and the New World, they found groups of people who painted themselves in bright and distinctive designs—a practice the explorers found unusual. The Europeans associated these customs with savagery and set about "civilizing" the "savages" by teaching them to stop using body paint and to start wearing European-style clothing.

Body paint was also used to protect the skin. The ancient Egyptians were devoted users of cosmetics. Their dramatic style of makeup included a preference for richly colored eyelids and thick, black

Thutu was an Egyptian noblewoman who lived in the thirteenth century B.C. Her beauty case, on display at the British Museum in London, shows how seriously she and other Egyptian women took their beauty rituals. Inside it were special slippers and elbow cushions for her comfort. She had pumice stones to remove body hair, as well as to smooth her elbows, knees, and feet. Little alabaster pots held her perfumes, face creams, and body creams. There were also ivory eye pencils for applying makeup to protect her eyes from the sun.

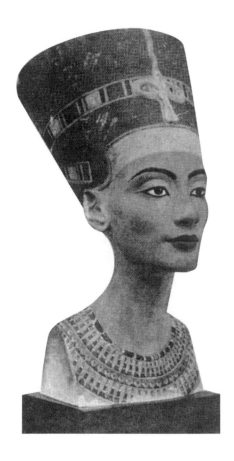

A bust of Queen Nefertiti (fourteenth century B.C.), illustrating the richly lined eyes and elaborate, head-dress-like hairstyles favored by ancient Egyptians

eyeliner. The cosmetic practices of the Egyptians may have made their appearances pleasing, but one of the primary reasons they used such thick paint on their eyes was for protection against the glaring Egyptian sun.

Some scholars believe Chinese women were the first to wear cosmetics for the sole purpose of making themselves more beautiful. In the thirteenth century in the southern regions of China, near Hangzhou, women used a white powder called *meen-fung* on their faces. They also used carmine, a bright red dye, on their cheeks, lips, and even inside their nostrils. They carefully plucked their eyebrows and

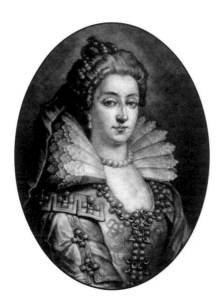

Like many other nobles of the day, Queen Elizabeth I (1533-1603) "sweetened" her breath with rinses made of sugar and wine, dyed her hair, and painted her face white.

cold cream: a cream used for cleaning and softening the skin

redrew them with a pencil or a piece of charcoal. Once the makeup was applied, they dusted their faces with rice powder to set it and soften the overall look.

TRENDSETTER QUEEN ELIZABETH I

During the time Queen Elizabeth I ruled England in the late 1500s, the use of cosmetics became very common. The queen set the standard, and women of the court followed her lead: dying their hair, plucking their eyebrows, and painting their faces. Some of the creams and lotions available to sixteenth-century women were actually harmful. A product called Soliman's Water, intended to remove freckles and warts, was made from mercury and was extremely poisonous. Women who used Soliman's Water regularly ruined both their skin and their health.

Women had traditionally passed on their knowledge of herbs and roots by word of mouth, but by the seventeenth century, some of those who could write were recording their secrets. They documented information about favorite recipes, cures for various illnesses, and preparations for clearing up the complexion. Eventually there were books available with information and ingredients for products such as tooth powder and cold cream. Women whose mothers or sisters had not passed on family formulas could now use these books to make their own products.

THE NEW WORLD

The practice of using makeup for beauty may have begun in China, but it also existed across the ocean among people unknown to Europeans until the fifteenth century. When the Spanish arrived in the New World, they began a process that led to a blending of different beauty traditions. The first Spanish adventurers met native Caribbean people who adorned their bodies with paint and feathers. In South America, the pre-Incan people of Peru used face powder and lip color. In what is now Mexico, Aztec women used a cosmetic called *axim* to improve their skin, and jojoba oil to condition their hair.

jojoba: a shrub with leathery leaves and edible seeds, which contain an oil commonly used in cosmetics and also as a lubricant

Early English settlers in America brought their own beauty recipes with them and blended them with those of Native Americans, African slaves, and other Europeans such as the French and Spanish. American Indians introduced them to plants that grew only in the Americas. African slaves brought traditions from their homelands in West Africa, such as smoothing their hair with grease and painting their cheeks with crushed berries.

THE STIGMA OF PAINTING

Mid- to late-nineteenth-century Western society had strict conventions about men and women's roles. Instead of working on the family farm as they had in past centuries, many men now worked outside their homes. Women ran the household, and their behavior impacted their husbands' reputations. Wives were expected to be virtuous, dressing modestly at all times. Misbehavior on their part threatened their family's social standing, so women were careful to monitor their own behavior even in the area of cosmetics use.

In the nineteenth century, a woman's appearance was often equated to her virtue. Pale, blemish-free skin, blushing cheeks, and expressive eyes were considered beautiful. If a woman were virtuous, then naturally her moral qualities would be reflected in her face. Women who used commercial products to alter their appearance were, at best, considered vain and artificial. At worst, they were called prostitutes or "Jezebels."

Women of that time, however, could use homemade recipes and traditional methods to improve their complexions naturally. These products, considered "cosmetics," were contrasted with "paints"—primarily commercial substances used to cover the skin. The line between the two was thin, though, and women were cautious not to cross it. Painting and powdering one's skin to conceal blemishes was dangerous and unethical; using cosmetics to improve the skin's quality was not.

As products became available through local drugstores, manufacturers began calling their products "cosmetics" instead of "paints" to blur the line between what was appropriate and what was not. Some women, however, were still uncomfortable about publicly purchasing cosmetics. Fortunately for these women, the publishing boom that occurred in the mid-nineteenth century gave them access to the information they needed to make their own skincare products.

The stigma associated with blemished skin led some women to "paint" in secret. One popular product on the market was called Laird's Bloom of

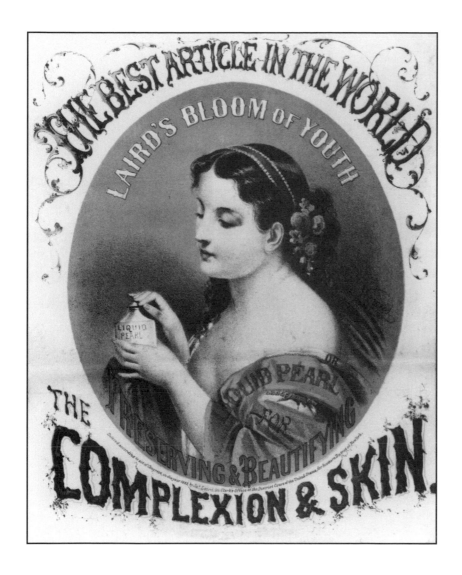

Youth. Advertisements claimed that women who used Laird's would have white skin, stay young-looking, and become popular because of both these benefits. Unfortunately, Laird's Bloom of Youth contained lead and could poison, even kill, women who used it on a regular basis. Women who wore Laird's Bloom of Youth and other products like it were often unwilling to admit it. Their silence

An early 1860s ad for Laird's Bloom of Youth "liquid pearl skin conditioner." The self-proclaimed "best article in the world," Laird's was made with lead and caused many women to become ill from using it.

increased the danger of using these products, because symptoms of lead poisoning were often misdiagnosed as hysterics or reproductive disorders.

Although cosmetics were available for purchase in the nineteenth century, there was no obvious "cosmetics industry." Women of this time who lived in or near big cities could purchase commercial items from their hairdressers and specialty stores. In the smaller cities and rural areas, women made their own products or bought them from sales agents who traveled all across the country peddling their goods.

Patent companies also began developing new cosmetics. The traditional use of the term "patent" stems from the practice of kings and queens in early modern Europe granting "patent rights" to individuals to encourage innovation. These were similar to the patents governments issue today, giving their holders the exclusive right to make certain products. In the nineteenth-century cosmetics business, however, the term "patent" was a generic name applied to all types of medicines and beauty products sold by a particular method of advertising and distribution.

By the 1800s, patent cosmetics companies had acquired a poor reputation. They were not required to list all the ingredients in their products, and a number of fashionable ones used dangerous substances like mercury, lead, or even arsenic. What gave patent companies their edge was convenience. They advertised directly to their customers using handbills, trade cards, or almanacs. They also guaranteed privacy by sending their orders wrapped in brown paper.

Theron Pond started Pond's, his patent remedy company, in 1846. Not wanting to lose customers because of the bad reputation patent companies were getting, he reorganized it as a beauty business in the 1890s. Now known as Chesebrough-Pond's, the company is still in business today.

Cosmetics in the Twentieth Century

Women in the early years of the twentieth century were still guided by their mothers' rules, but change was on the way. Proper attire remained somewhat stiff and structured, but undergarment styles were looser with fewer corsets. Entertaining was formal and frequent, but women were also getting involved in sports and outdoor activities. They still wore very little colored cosmetics on their faces, biting their lips or pinching their cheeks to add color during the day. In the evening, however, they went so far as to use berries or pure vegetable food coloring on their lips for color, and some women and girls from respectable families occasionally appeared in public wearing powder and rouge on their cheeks. This was still risky for a woman's reputation in the early 1900s, however, as overtly "making up" one's face was still considered an activity primarily for actors and prostitutes. In 1913, one saleswoman for Macy's found out just how risky the practice was when she was fired after coming to work with rouged cheeks. Her manager announced, "[I am] not running a theatrical troupe but a department store."

Change was likely, however, as more and more women started working in offices or stores. For many of these women, the growing beauty business was a chance to earn a good living while doing something they enjoyed. These early workers in the beauty business served as beauty culturists or cosmeticians. Working out of storefronts similar to hair salons, they gave skin treatments to customers,

In 1914, George Bunting made a concoction to soothe sunburn and eczema (a skin condition characterized by itching, redness, and scaly patches). He sold the cream to women vacationing along Maryland's beaches, claiming it could "knock eczema." The phrase stuck, and the product became known as "Noxzema." Bunting eventually promoted it nationally as an inexpensive facial cleanser and moisturizer. By the twenty-first century, Noxzema came in 13 varieties and was sold all over the world.

rouge: a type of cosmetic, usually red or pink in color, applied to the lips or cheeks

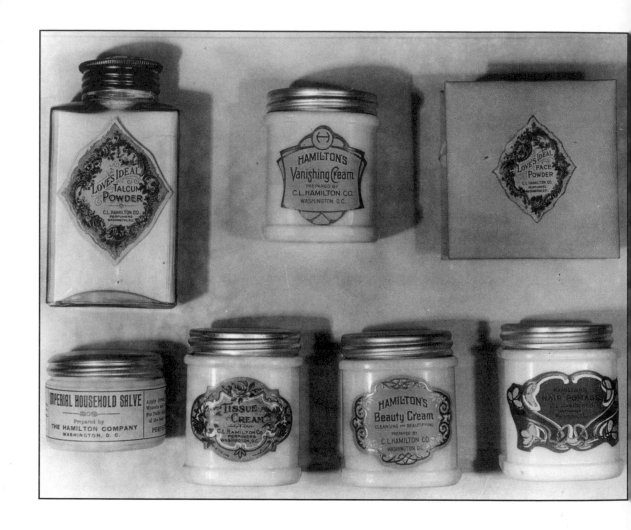

Some of the "acceptable" cosmetic products available in the early years of the twentieth century included hair pomade, talcum powder, and cold cream. By the 1920s, many companies, such as Hamilton, had begun developing complete lines of these products intended for use together.

massaging lotions into the skin to keep it healthy. It soon became obvious to these pioneers in the beauty industry that they could add to their income by selling, right in their salons, the products they used on their customers' faces They eventually took their businesses a step further by developing complete sets of creams and lotions designed for use with one another.

WOMAN'S WORK

Women who wanted, or needed, to work in the late nineteenth and early twentieth centuries had few options. Only certain jobs, such as typing, sales, sewing, nursing, or teaching were considered appropriate for women. Being forced to work in certain fields limited their chances for advancement, but the beauty industry provided the perfect opportunity for ambitious women to build successful businesses. Women had always traded beauty secrets and taken care of each other's hair and skin, so it was not a big step for a woman to open a hair or beauty salon. Ambitious women could, for money, do exactly what they had been doing at home with their sisters and daughters. They did not need traditional methods of advertising to help their businesses grow—once a woman liked what she experienced in the salon, she would spread the word to her family and friends. This style of advertising built on patterns in women's social lives.

Not only did the beauty industry create a good opportunity for women to become financially independent, but it was also perfect for female immigrants or ethnic minorities, who had even fewer employment prospects than other women. Some of the first women to build successful beauty businesses were from groups outside the mainstream of society. Helena Rubinstein was an immigrant with very little money when she started her business in Australia, and Madam C. J. Walker was an African American daughter of former slaves.

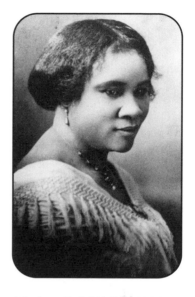

Madam C. J. Walker (1867-1919), creator of Wonderful Hair Grower, turned her mail-order business into an empire, becoming the first African American female millionaire. Wanting to give others like herself a chance for success, Walker traveled the country recruiting and training black women as sales agents. She also founded Lelia College, a sales training school exclusively for Walker agents.

Madam C. J. Walker

Sarah Breedlove's childhood was not an easy one. It was hard enough being born black in the South in 1867, but she also had the misfortune of losing both her parents by the time she was six years old. An older sister took her in after she was orphaned. She married Moses McWilliams when she was just 14. Misfortune struck again when Breedlove was widowed before she turned 20. In 1888, she moved to St. Louis with her baby daughter, Lelia, and found work washing clothes and cleaning houses.

Soon after, Breedlove noticed her hair was beginning to fall out. But instead of being ashamed of her problem, she decided to do something about it. Over the years, she experimented with various hair products, trying to find a formula that would help her hair grow back. Her persistence paid off when she developed a product that not only stimulated hair to grow, but also actually gave it a healthy glow. Breedlove called her miracle product the "Wonderful Hair Grower." She knew from talking to her friends that she was not the only black woman with hair problems, and she thought her product could help them as well. She practiced applying the hair grower to her own hair, brushing it until it shone, and then using a hot comb to smooth and style it. She was amazed at the results, and the process eventually came to be known as the "Walker System." (Sarah had married Charles J. Walker in 1906.)

Whenever she could find the time between working and caring for her family, Walker took her hair grower door-to-door, demonstrating to other African American women how healthy and beautiful she could make their hair look. The Wonderful Hair Grower became so popular she was soon recruiting "Walker agents" to sell it.

With her business a success, Walker was able to give up the menial jobs that had helped her survive. She began calling herself "Madam C. J." Walker, and she and her family moved to Denver, then Indianapolis, where she focused her energies on manufacturing her product and training women who were clamoring to become Walker agents. She kept up a hectic pace, traveling from state to state, training agents to use her hair-care system, and selling her product.

During the early years of the twentieth century, traveling across the country was a daring feat for any woman, and even more so for a black woman. At the time there was still a high level of prejudice against blacks, and lynchings were not uncommon. But Walker's dreams of success spurred her on. In addition to spending countless hours on the road, Walker made sure her company name was recognized. She placed advertisements in as many black newspapers, farm journals, and religious periodicals as she could. Her bravery and willingness to work hard paid off, and at one point her company was the largest black-owned business in the entire country, employing around 3,000 people.

In 1919, Walker introduced skin-care products and face powders. She wanted to help women like herself, who had not grown up feeling beautiful, to look their best. Her goal was not for black women to emulate the Caucasian standard of beauty, but to help them highlight the best in their African features. She believed beauty had nothing to do with skin color and refused to sell skin bleach to her customers as others had done.

Some influential people in the black community criticized Walker for selling cosmetics, which they considered disreputable and even sinful. But she thought the self-esteem black women developed from using her products and working as Walker agents made her business a vital one.

After Walker's death in 1919, her general manager, F. B. Ransom, took over the running of the company. In spite of Walker's philosophies, Ransom made changes to the product line, including introducing a skin bleach called Tan-Off. Ironically, sales for Tan-Off soon outpaced those for the original product "Wonderful Hair Grower." In 1985, the company was sold by the trustees of the Walker estate and is no longer in business today.

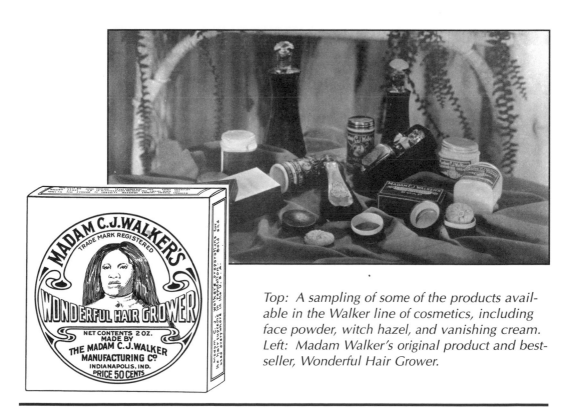

Top: A sampling of some of the products available in the Walker line of cosmetics, including face powder, witch hazel, and vanishing cream. Left: Madam Walker's original product and bestseller, Wonderful Hair Grower.

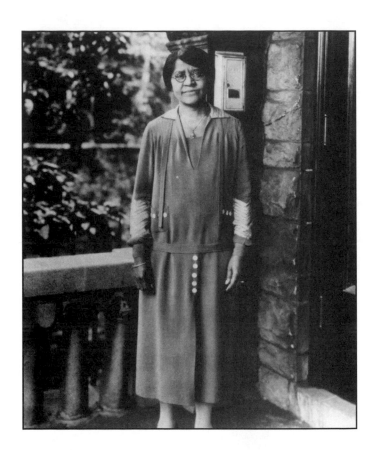

A contemporary and former employer of Madam C. J. Walker, Annie Turnbo Malone (1869-1957) also made her fortune selling beauty products for African American women. Her Poro line of hair-care products was an international success, and many credit it with being the inspiration for Walker's Wonderful Hair Grower. "Poro" is a West African term that refers to an organization that disciplines and enhances a person's spirit and physical body.

THE ETHNIC MARKET

It would be well into the 1970s before major cosmetics companies began making serious efforts to respond to African American women's needs. Two of the earliest success stories in the beauty business, however, feature black women: Madam C. J. Walker, and Annie Turnbo Malone. Walker and Malone built their businesses catering to African American women's hair care. They filled a huge void by helping these women clean, condition, and style their hair, and they also made the conscious decision to structure their businesses to create jobs for black women.

Not all the early marketers of beauty products for African Americans were concerned about helping them. Some reinforced stereotypes that implied beauty meant light skin. These marketers offered skin lighteners, or "black skin removers," that promised to give African American women "peach-like" complexions.

In the late 1950s and 1960s, African American models began to appear in advertising, but they were the exceptions instead of the rule. In 1974, *Vogue* magazine took a bold step by featuring an African American model, Beverly Johnson, on its cover. It

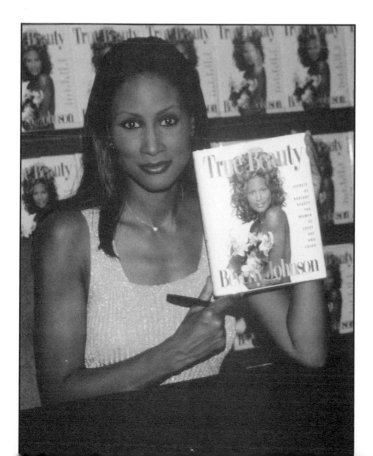

Beverly Johnson's success as an international cover model gave her the chance to pursue other opportunities, such as singing, acting, and writing. Here, Johnson conducts a book signing for her autobiography, True Beauty.

was the first time a mainstream magazine had done this—indicating that the needs of women of color were finally being addressed. Until then, most African American women had been making do with whatever cosmetics they could find or devise. According to Susan L. Taylor, editorial director of *Essence* magazine, "We mixed and stirred and blended Avon and Chanel with cocoa powder or ground cinnamon and Crisco." But during the 1970s some cosmetics companies brought out lines specifically for the African American market. One company, Avon, added a wider range of foundation shades and makeup colors to its existing lines instead of creating separate lines for women of color. This proved to be a brilliant decision, because it allowed African American women to purchase cosmetics designed for them without being singled out. Avon also hired African American sales agents to help sell the company's products.

THE BUSINESS OF COSMETICS

Even though the cosmetics business started as a female-dominated occupation, by the 1920s men had moved into the industry. Before World War I, the beauty business was local and service-oriented, and women took care of women, setting up schools to teach beauty systems and offering their students franchise opportunities. But during the same period in which female-operated businesses were growing, new business methods were developing, and a group of male business professionals emerged. Instead of small-scale production methods, a national system

franchise: a licensing arrangement in which an investor pays money to the owner of a particular brand-name product or business for permission to sell that product or operate that business in a certain territory. The person offering the permission is called the **franchiser**. The person buying the rights is the **franchisee**.

of mass production developed, and products were distributed, marketed, and advertised in new ways.

Men such as Carl Weeks, founder of Armand, played a major role in developing the mass market for the beauty business. Weeks started his career as a drugstore owner. He began experimenting with face powder by trying to make a product that would last longer than others on the market. He packaged

mass production: the manufacture of goods in large quantities

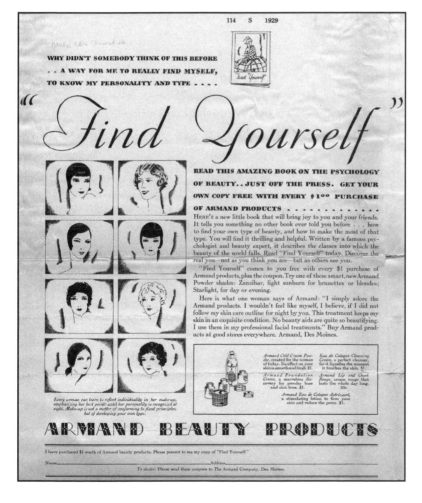

Armand's 1929 "Find Yourself" advertising campaign featured more than 30 different types of women and encouraged women to pick the one they most identified with. These panels show a selection of "types" from one of the ads.

his powder in a tiny version of a hatbox, hoping customers would get the impression of Parisian chic. Weeks focused on building a distribution network to get his product efficiently to the drugstores that carried it. He also gave away free powder samples, designed window displays, and wrote newsletters full of sales advice. From 1912 until 1927, Armand grew from a business with $5,000 in annual sales to one with $2.5 million, all based on face powder. During the Great Depression, however, sales dropped because few women had money to spend on cosmetics. Tired of heavy face powders, women also started to buy lighter powders from other companies, and Armand's business declined. In 1949, Weeks resigned from Armand and the company was merged with one that he and his brothers owned called the D. C. Weeks Company. The new company, Weeks & Leo, sold over-the-counter medicines and some toiletries such as lotions and creams. Weeks died in 1962.

ADVERTISING BOOM

As the way of doing business changed in the twentieth century, so did advertising techniques. Ads were designed to appeal to women, many of whom were now working and had their own money to spend. Advertising firms created departments devoted to studying the buying habits of consumers and developed campaigns to take advantage of this information. Before 1918, advertising for cosmetics was limited, but a period of phenomenal growth occurred between 1915 and about 1930. Money spent on magazine advertising rose from $1.3 million to $16 million. Many business owners turned to using one of the new advertising firms to be competitive. Even Carl Weeks, who had excellent marketing instincts, hired a New York advertising firm to develop a national campaign for Armand.

Before corporations dominated the cosmetics business, dynamic individuals had created the industry with their own drive to succeed. Some, like Helena Rubinstein, Elizabeth Arden, and Estée Lauder, used similar techniques to get their businesses started. Others—like David Hall McConnell of Avon, who started as a door-to-door salesman—found their own unique paths into the beauty business. Charles Revson of Revlon made copying other business leaders an art, while Anita Roddick challenged the corporate world with her unconventional approach to making and selling beauty products.

The cosmetics industry continues to be a dominant force in the economy while eliciting both praise and criticism for its effect on our society. However they are viewed, cosmetics use and the business supporting it are both permanent parts of our culture, and they are likely to be so for years to come.

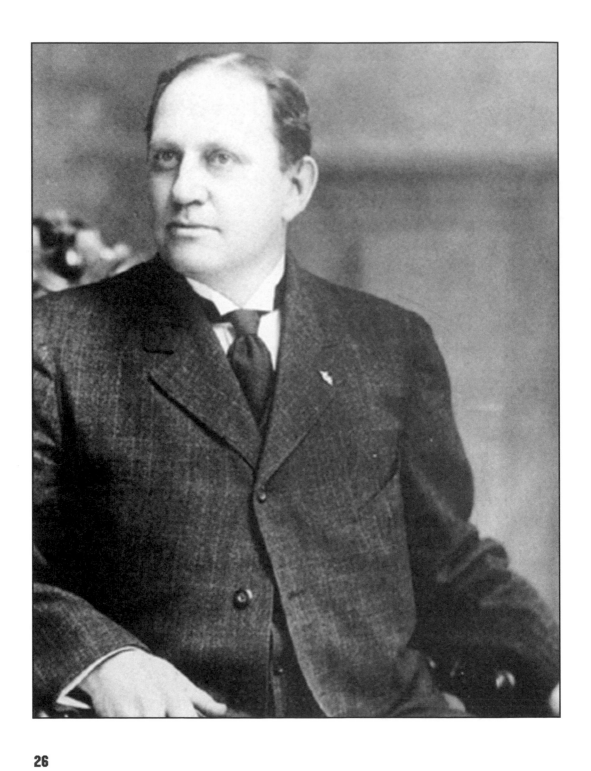

1

DAVID MCCONNELL

AVON PRODUCTS:
ONE DOOR AT A TIME

David McConnell looked over his books and carefully reviewed his sales dialogue. He had been selling books for years, but he wanted to be sure his delivery was smooth and his manner friendly when he made his presentation. Today would be different, because in addition to books, he would also take a few sample bottles of perfume to offer to his customers. He hoped the perfume would pique the women's interest and help him sell his books, but he soon found the perfume idea was a success in a way he had not anticipated. After a few weeks of trying to use the fragrances to help increase book sales, McConnell realized that his customers were not very interested in adding to their libraries, but they were enthusiastic about his perfume. If perfume was what

David Hall McConnell (1858-1937) used his talent and knowledge as a door-to-door salesman to found the California Perfume Company, a business that would grow to become Avon, the largest direct-sales cosmetics company in the world.

they wanted, that was what he would give them. In the mid-1880s, the door-to-door book salesman became a supplier of perfume.

BECOMING A BUSINESS OWNER

David Hall McConnell was born on July 18, 1858, in Oswego, New York, the son of Irish immigrants James McConnell and Isabel Hall. After he finished school, he planned to become a mathematics teacher, but instead, in 1879, he began selling books for a company that specialized in door-to-door sales. Though he never really loved the job, he did well. After three years, he was put in charge of the southern territory, which required him to move to Atlanta, Georgia. After doing so well as a salesman, McConnell realized teaching mathematics was not in his future. Instead, he began dreaming of having his own company.

With this goal in mind, he committed himself to learning all he could about direct sales and to looking for a business opportunity. He did not have to wait long. When his boss decided to sell his business, McConnell jumped at the opportunity to purchase it. Now he was a business owner, but he knew he did not want to continue selling only books. He needed a product he could sell directly to his customers, one that would be consumed so he would have a built-in repeat business. Methodically he researched and eliminated various products until he came up with the idea of making a perfume. Women loved perfume and if they liked a particular scent, they would buy it over and over again. He shared his idea with

direct sales: the sale of goods from one individual to another, often done door-to-door or in the customer's home. Avon products and Girl Scout cookies are examples of products sold by direct sales.

Lucy, his wife, and they decided perfume might be the product they could use to expand their business.

THE CALIFORNIA PERFUME COMPANY

First, David McConnell read everything he could find about making perfume. He and Lucy then experimented with different scents until they found something they thought might be popular, and he started taking free samples of the scent with him on his sales trips. By 1886, McConnell was confident enough about selling perfumes that he founded the California Perfume Company. In spite of its name, the California Perfume Company was always based in New York. McConnell chose the name because of the glowing reports he received about California in letters from his former employer. David and Lucy continued experimenting with fragrances in the company's first office, an old warehouse near Wall Street in New York City. When they had five fragrances, they put them together in a set and called it the Little Dot Perfume Set. The collection included scents they had decided were winners: Violet, White Rose, Heliotrope, Lily-of-the-Valley, and Hyacinth.

Now that he had a product, McConnell needed someone to sell it, and he had the perfect person in mind. Parshis Foster Eames Albee already worked for McConnell, and he knew she would be perfect for selling perfumes to other women. When he approached her about his idea to transition the business out of bookselling and into perfumes, she was as excited as he was. She came up with a plan not only to canvass her neighborhood selling perfumes, but

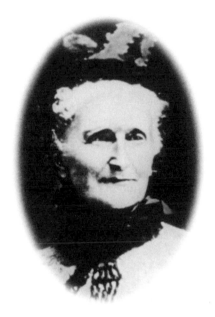

One of McConnell's most successful bookselling agents was Parshis F. E. Albee. When McConnell could no longer handle the California Perfume Company's sales volume alone, she was the first agent he hired. Considered the first "Avon Lady," Albee was such a successful businesswoman that in 1997 a Barbie doll was created in her honor.

also to recruit other women to do the same in their neighborhoods. The job would allow women to earn a little money of their own while working around their families' schedules.

Confident in his choice for the California Perfume Company's first saleswoman, McConnell handed Albee his sample case, turned over the day-to-day operations to her, and set about building his product line. Albee was his only salesperson in the first six months of business, but she soon built a sales team of women who worked part-time. Using a female sales force gave an air of friendliness and gentility to the company image, but it also accomplished something else—an opportunity to expand beyond perfumes into the toiletries market. A woman who might not make a special trip to a store to purchase these products would be happy to try toiletries brought to her door by a friendly saleswoman. McConnell knew these products could be successfully added to his line in the future.

ADDING TO THE LINE: AVON PRODUCTS

With Albee taking care of sales, the perfume orders increased and David and Lucy could no longer meet the demand in their small space. Besides, their family was growing and Lucy needed to take care of their three children: Edna Bertha, Dorys Hall, and David Hall Jr. In 1897, David decided to open a perfume laboratory near their home in Suffern, New York, and to expand the product line. Along with perfumes, he created toiletries such as shampoo, witch hazel cream, and toothpaste. Later he added

toiletries: articles used in personal grooming, such as toothpaste and hair spray

witch hazel: a solution made from the bark and leaves of the witch hazel shrub and used as an astringent

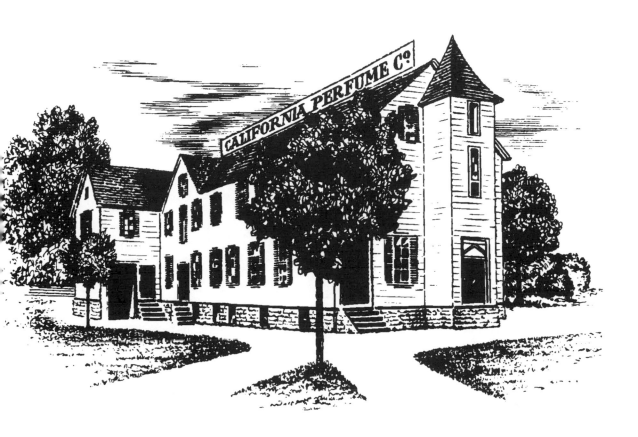

household articles such as flavoring extracts and sold them under the brand name Perfection. Perfumes remained the base of his business, but McConnell realized that the company had grown too big for him to devote sufficient attention to their manufacturing—he needed to hire a professional. Adolf Goetting had been in business for 25 years and was the top perfumer of his day. In order to hire him, McConnell bought out Goetting's business and laboratory.

Because the California Perfume Company sold its products door-to-door from the very first day,

McConnell used this sketch of the California Perfume Company's new factory in Suffern, New York, on the cover of his autobiography, Great Oak. *The picture was drawn just after the factory opened for production in 1897.*

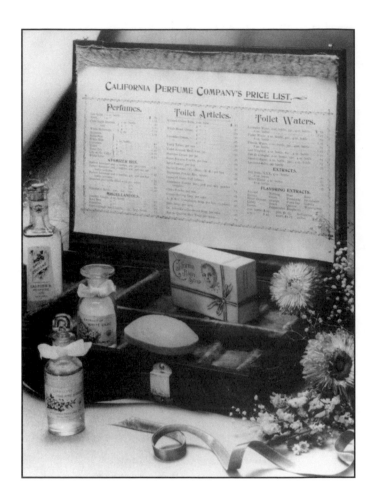

As of the early 1920s, Avon (then still called the California Perfume Company) had not yet tapped into the new color-cosmetic market. This sales case shows items for sale in the late 1910s and early 1920s, including baby soap, perfumes, shampoo, and witch hazel extract.

McConnell paid special attention to his shipping department. He knew there was potential for the company's image to be tarnished by poorly packed products, and he was also aware of the disappointment and frustration customers would feel if their order arrived with items missing. He made a special effort to maintain excellence in this department and was proud to write in his 1903 autobiography, "Each order is handled as though it is the only order to be shipped."

In 1906, the California Perfume Company placed its first print ads, in *Good Housekeeping* magazine, as well as issued its first full-color catalog. By January 1916, the California Perfume Company had been in business for 30 years and was doing so well the McConnells decided to incorporate it. Sales surpassed the $1 million mark in 1920, and reached $2 million by 1926. In 1928, twelve years after incorporating, the company introduced a line of cosmetics and toiletries called Avon. McConnell chose this name after a friend visited Stratford-upon-Avon, William Shakespeare's birthplace in England, and

Avon was a family business, and all of the McConnell children were actively involved in the company, as well as in the charitable organizations it helped fund. Here, David McConnell Sr. poses with his son, David Jr., who would succeed his father as Avon's president.

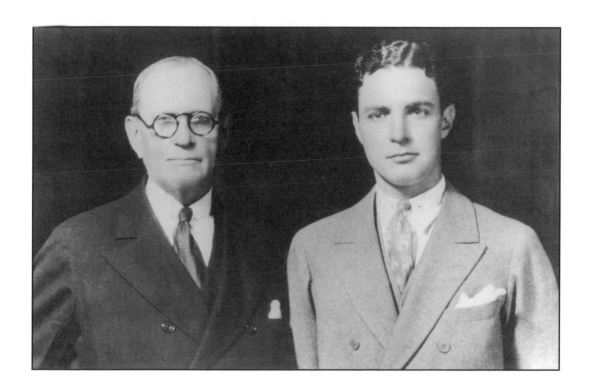

was struck by how similar the countryside was to the landscape around the California Perfume Company's headquarters. The name became so popular that in 1939, McConnell's son David Jr., who had succeeded his father as president, changed the company's name to Avon.

Like the product line, the sales force Albee trained grew. By 1903 there were more than 10,000 salespeople selling the company's products.

Avon took out its first magazine ad in 1906. By 1957, when this advertisement was published, Avon had full-color ads in publications that reached an audience of more than 50 million women annually.

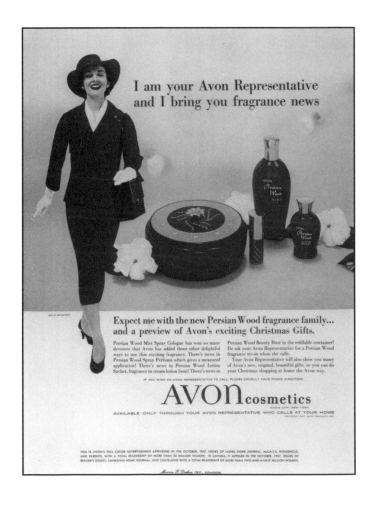

Independent representatives, as they later came to be called, gave their customers personal service by providing catalogs filled with color pictures of the company's growing line of products. By 1937, the number of independent representatives had increased to more than 30,000.

In addition to his positions as president, chairman of the board, and principal owner of Avon Products, Inc., which he held until his death, McConnell kept active in his community. At various times he was treasurer of G. W. Carnrick and Co., manufacturers of pharmaceutical supplies in Newark, New Jersey; a director of the Holly Hill Fruit Products, Inc., an orange grove and canning enterprise in Davenport, Florida; one of the founders of the Suffern National Bank and later president and chairman of the board; superintendent of schools in Suffern; and president of the Suffern Board of Education. He also played an important part in building the Suffern Presbyterian Church. As active as he was, he still found time to pursue his hobbies: fishing, golf, and horseback riding.

LEGACY

David McConnell died in Suffern, New York, on January 20, 1937, leaving behind a company with a sales volume already in the millions. By 2002, Avon had annual sales of $6 billion and employed 3.5 million sales representatives. The company marketed its own brands of makeup, skin-care and hair-care items, fragrances, jewelry, clothing, and more. Avon was also a generous contributor to charitable causes.

After McConnell's death, his son-in-law, Van Alan Clark, who was married to Edna McConnell, continued to work at Avon and became chairman of the board in the 1950s. The Clarks created a foundation that offered grants to help children, the poor, the elderly, and the developing world. Avon's Worldwide Fund for Women's Health raised close to $200 million in the 10 years following its creation in 1992. Avon also led the way in creating awareness of breast cancer. In 1993, the company introduced its "pink ribbon" products, which helped raise funds to fight the disease. The first Avon Breast Cancer 3-Day Walk took place in southern California five years later. In addition, Avon donated $250,000 in honor of the company's fragrance Women of the World to the Avon Breast Cancer Awareness Crusade.

In 2000, tennis stars Venus and Serena Williams signed on as spokespersons for Avon products through the company's "Let's Talk" advertising campaign. In 2001, Avon broadened its marketing focus and entered the retail market, targeting women who preferred to shop in stores and who were not already customers through the direct-selling channel. The line of products, beComing, was marketed through J. C. Penney department stores across the country. This venture into retail did not reduce Avon's direct appeal, and the company still held the position of being the foremost direct seller of beauty products in the world. While being known for such staples as perfumes and lotions, the company also built a reputation for taking advantage of the newest technology and advances in understanding skin biology.

retail: selling goods in small amounts directly to customers. Wal-Mart and Target are examples of retail stores.

In the early 1990s, through its Anew line, Avon became the first company to market a skin-care product that made use of alpha-hydroxy acid technology to help keep skin looking young. Each year, Avon also produced a new perfume made up of scents from around the globe. Two of these fragrances, Women of the Earth, introduced in 1998, and Perceive, in 1999, set records for best-selling

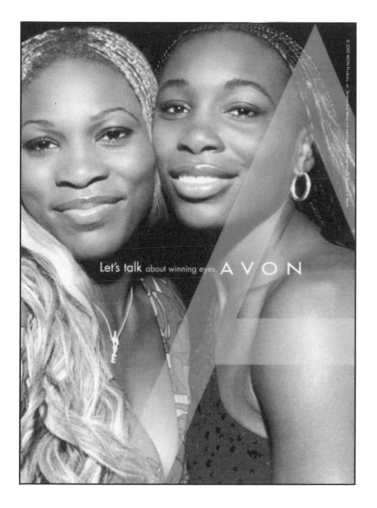

Let's talk about winning eyes. A V O N

One of the reasons Avon chose Venus and Serena Williams as spokespeople for its "Let's Talk" campaign was because of the sisters' commitment to health and fitness. The company also encouraged women to be active in many other ways. For example, it sponsored several three-day walks for breast cancer research across the country each year. Avon also founded the Avon Running Global Circuit, a series of women-only 10-kilometer races. Local women competed in a regional race, and winners advanced to race at the national, and then world-wide, championships.

fragrance launches in the world. Perceive made use of cutting-edge technology: synthesized human pheromones (chemicals that send messages to the brain through the sense of smell). Perceive's synthesized pheromones were created to help the woman wearing the fragrance feel more positive. Another Avon toiletry, Skin-So-Soft body lotion, became so well known for repelling mosquitoes that the company produced a version specifically for use as a mosquito repellent. Future plans included a product line designed for menopausal women.

In 1886, when McConnell first founded the California Perfume Company, he dreamed of running his own business and giving his customers the best quality products he could. He was aware of his company's potential when, in 1903, he wrote, "As the California Perfume Company's business has grown in the past, so shall it grow in the future; the limit in this business is measured only by the amount of hard work and energy that you and I put in it."

When David McConnell turned to Parshis Albee for help in running his company, he set a precedent for creating an environment where women could realize their professional dreams in a nurturing environment. According to Andrea Jung, the company's chief executive officer and chairman of the board, there is no glass ceiling at Avon. Avon became one of the most widely recognized companies in the world and a leading advocate of women's issues. It also set the standard for countless direct-selling companies that continue to emerge both inside and outside the cosmetics industry.

Avon has more women in management positions than any other Fortune 500 company (86 percent). Half of the members of its board of directors are female.

The term "glass ceiling" refers to unacknowledged discrimination that keeps women and minorities from rising to positions of power in major industries and companies.

Mary Kay Cosmetics

When Mary Kay Ash died in 2001, she left behind hundreds of beauty consultants, sales directors, and national sales directors committed to marketing her products with the "go-give" (the more you go out and give, the more you receive in return) spirit she developed.

Ash started her company in Dallas, Texas, in 1963, after retiring from a career in sales. Her venture actually began as she was writing a training guide for career women. In this book, she listed all the things she thought made up the ideal company. In her own career, she had encountered many obstacles to success because she was a woman, and she brainstormed to find ways women could excel in this fictional company. By the time her outline for the book was finished, she realized she had a blueprint for a successful business—what she needed was a product.

For years Ash had been using cosmetics developed by a friend whose father was a tanner (someone who turns raw animal skins into leather), and she felt his products would be perfect for her to build her company around. She purchased the original formulas from the tanner's heirs and started Mary Kay Cosmetics.

Rather than selling her products in retail outlets, Ash decided to sell them in a relaxing environment where women could try the products before they made their purchases. She recruited others who, like herself, would go into homes and give demonstrations to groups of women. From the beginning, the goal was to empower women instead of just selling makeup. Consultants were encouraged to have a giving attitude by helping each other to build successful businesses. The fact that Ash's creams and lotions were good for the skin was almost an extra bonus.

Ash instituted a reward system offering jewelry and fur coats and unlimited promotion opportunities for her beauty consultants. The company's top directors drove distinctive pink Cadillacs and many enjoyed lucrative salaries. Another reward offered was the jeweled bumblebee pin. Many scientists have said that a bee shouldn't be able to fly—its wings are too small for its body—but it does. Ash felt the bumblebee was a good symbol for her and other representatives because they succeeded when others thought they could not.

In addition to the basic skin-care system for the face, in 2003, Mary Kay Cosmetics offered body-care items, men's skin care, fragrances, and a full line of color cosmetics. The company remained committed to the personal touch direct selling allows.

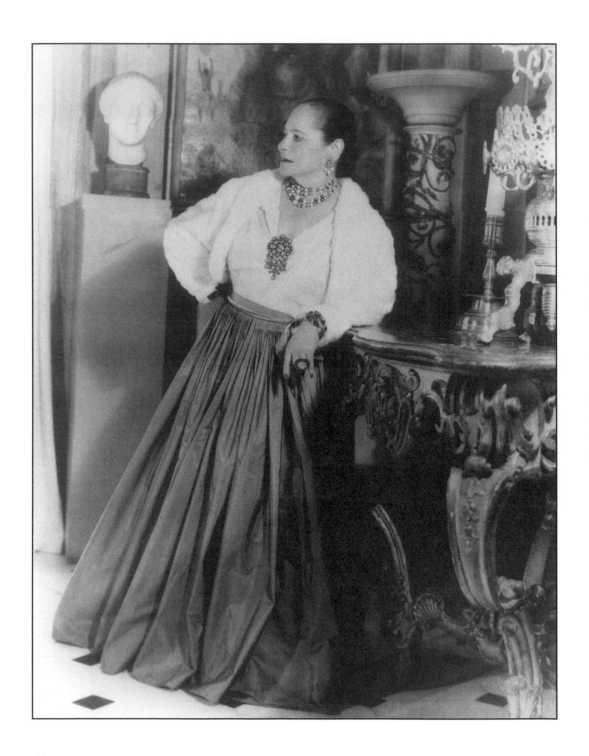

2

HELENA RUBINSTEIN

INNOVATING BEAUTY

In 1915, Helena Rubinstein arrived in New York City. After living and working in some of the world's most exciting cities, she thought New York seemed a logical next step for her. With interest, she noticed the city's women and knew she had made the right decision to move to New York. "All the American women had purple noses and gray lips, and their faces were chalk white from terrible powder," she said. "I recognized that the United States could be my life's work."

Rubinstein was not a struggling immigrant when she first came to the United States. She had successful beauty salons in Paris, London, and Melbourne, Australia. But in America, she would rise to the top of the beauty industry with her innovations in beauty culture. She would also test her

Polish-born Helena Rubinstein (1870?-1965) was both an innovator and a shrewd judge of talent. Many of her products were self-created, but many others she found by "ferret[ing] out 'clever novelties'" and then paying the inventors an annual royalty for the rights to merchandise their products.

mettle against rival Elizabeth Arden, whose every move she would be aware of—even though the two never met.

GOOD SKIN, GOOD BUSINESS

The details of the early years of Helena Rubinstein's life are hazy. She was born in Cracow, Poland, on December 25, sometime in the early 1870s, the eldest of eight girls. Her father was in the wholesale food trade and, although the family was not wealthy, they lived comfortably. Around the age of 18, Helena decided she wanted to marry a young medical student from a nearby university. Her father disapproved of this and wanted her to marry someone else, so to escape her situation she decided to visit an uncle who lived in Australia. In around 1889 (although it may have been earlier), she packed her bags, boarded a ship, and left home for a new life.

As luck would have it, her move to Australia meant that instead of being one of many young girls in Cracow with beautiful skin, she stood out in the tough Australian climate, where women had sun-damaged and wind-hardened skin. Helena and her sisters had been using a face cream made by a family friend, a chemist named Dr. Jacob Lykusky. In preparation for Helena's journey, her mother packed 12 pots of the cream so Helena would be able to continue taking good care of her skin. While she lived with her uncle, she shared her face cream with the women she met. Inspired by their interest in her skin care routine, Helena asked Lykusky to send more cream. This time, she decided to use the

There is some debate about the actual year of Helena Rubinstein's birth, as well as when exactly she opened up her first few shops. She preferred to keep that information secret, and when asked about her past she would frequently refuse to respond, saying, "What's the use of looking back?"

wholesale: selling goods in bulk, or in large quantities, usually done from the manufacturer to the retail store

cream to help her make a living and to leave the rural ranch where her uncle lived.

She had escaped her strict father's marriage decisions, but Helena Rubinstein was not happy staying with her uncle. She was living in Coleraine, a small sheep-ranching community about 80 miles away from Melbourne, where she really wanted to live. When a friend she had made on the voyage to Australia invited her to come to Melbourne and stay with her, Rubinstein went. With the security of a place to stay, and an idea for a business, Rubinstein settled in the city.

MAISON DE BEAUTÉ VALAZE

Rubinstein was always very vague about the years she spent in Melbourne, but her goal was to open her own business, and she eventually did.

Another friend Rubinstein had met on board the ship from Europe to Australia was Helen MacDonald. They stayed in touch, and when Rubinstein needed the money to start her business, MacDonald gave her a loan. Rubinstein had decided that in addition to selling her creams, she would open a shop where women could come to learn the techniques she used to keep her own skin healthy and beautiful. She wanted to create an elegant environment that would make a woman's visit a special experience she would want to repeat. With this in mind, she used her money carefully.

First, she ordered a large stock of cream from Lykusky in Poland. Without the cream she would have no business, so she made sure she had enough to handle the expected demand. Then she rented a second-floor room on a street in the heart of Melbourne, where her customers could easily reach her and where her shop would be noticed. Finally, she bought jars and labels. While waiting for her creams to arrive, Rubinstein gave special dramatic touches to her shop by adding rattan furniture and making curtains from the luxurious fabrics that were once the skirts of her dresses. By the time the cream arrived she had settled on a name for it, Valaze Russian Skin Food, and her shop would be called the Maison de Beauté Valaze.

An early ad (ca. 1905) for Valaze Skin Food. The ad was designed by Edward Titus and extolled the virtues and benefits of the cream. Rubinstein helped make creativity in advertising one of the hallmarks of the early cosmetics moguls. Although this ad seems simple, over the next few decades, campaigns grew more complex. For example, in the 1940s, Rubinstein launched a new fragrance, Heaven Sent, by floating hundreds of fragrance samples attached to pale blue balloons from the windows of her office down onto Fifth Avenue.

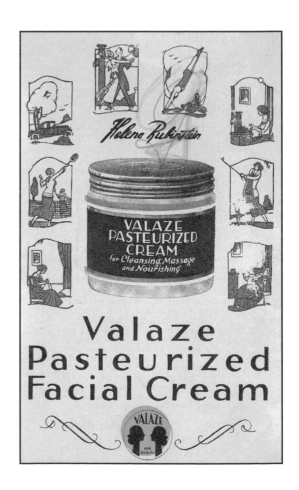

INNOVATIONS

With everything in place, Rubinstein opened her doors for business. It was 1904 and the beginning of a journey she could never have imagined. The Australian women flocked to her salon, and it wasn't long before she needed another shipment of cream from Poland. She convinced Lykusky, as well as two of her sisters, Manka and Ceska, to come to Australia and help her run the business.

Rubinstein had started her business with one cream, but she wanted Lykusky to create other products. In working with many different women, she noticed that each woman had a different skin type. Not only would Rubinstein need more products for normal skin like hers, but she would also have to develop different lines of products for other skin types. She grouped women's skin into four categories: oily, dry, combination, and normal. This was a completely new way of approaching skin care. Women in Europe had been used to cleansing their skin with a cold cream, but the idea of adjusting the products they used to match their type of skin was truly innovative.

Lykusky had taught Rubinstein and her sisters the beauty techniques they used on their own skin, and these were the techniques Rubinstein taught the women of Australia. First, she had them clean their faces with a cold cream instead of a harsh soap. She followed this with an astringent to close the pores and give a smooth appearance, and finally with a vanishing cream to moisturize and protect their skin.

astringent: a substance that causes tissues in the body to constrict or draw together

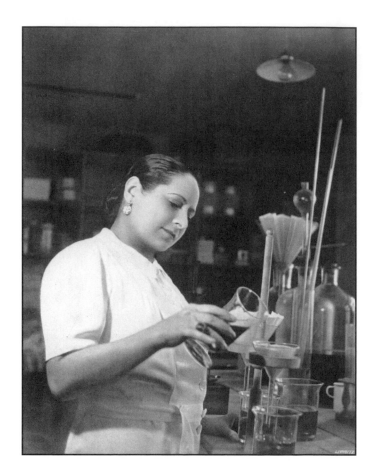

Although she initially had Lykusky make her creams, Rubinstein quickly took over their manufacture and development, often mixing the formulas herself. "I'm happiest working in my 'kitchen,'" she said.

Rubinstein took her business seriously and was determined to address the needs of her customers so they could have the beautiful skin they admired in her. Her focus led to another innovation. Noting that skin seemed to have different needs at different times of the day, she developed creams for the night that had different ingredients from those used during the day.

Her salon attracted enough attention to warrant an article in a Sydney, Australia, newspaper and more women demanded her creams. In addition to helping her shop, the article gave Rubinstein a marketing idea. If she could get a well-known person to use her products and talk about them, she would generate even more interest in her skin-care business. She recruited a famous opera singer, Nellie Melba, to promote the Valaze cream, and her idea paid off— Rubinstein was a success in Australia.

Shops in London and Paris

It is not clear exactly when Rubinstein moved to England, but sometime around 1908 she decided to leave her adopted homeland. Although she was doing well in Australia, there was little opportunity to expand her business in the sparsely populated country. Another reason she left was similar to the reason she went there in the first place: to avoid marriage. She had met an American writer named Edward Titus who wanted to get married, but she was just beginning to achieve real success and did not want to focus on romance. Rubinstein went to England without Titus, and told him to wait and see if her business was successful. Titus apparently followed her to England and they were married. The union, however, did not hold up as well as the business, and eventually the pair divorced. They had two sons, Roy and Horace, both of whom were involved in various aspects of Rubinstein's business for most of their lives.

In London, Rubinstein opened a new Maison de Beauté Valaze on Grafton Street in the heart of Mayfair, a popular and visible location. She was

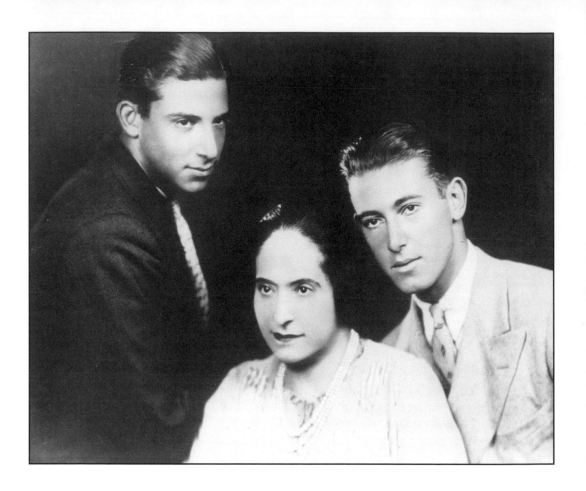

Rubinstein and her sons. Both Roy (left) and Horace (right) Titus were involved in the business throughout their lives.

soon able to attract many wealthy customers who endorsed her products. The success of her salon in London opened her eyes to the possibilities for launching new salons in other cities.

By 1912, Rubinstein was ready to launch yet another salon. Beauty treatments and beauty products had caught the attention of women around the world, and she believed there was a tremendous future for her in the fledgling industry. Rubinstein knew that Paris, the city whose royal court had dictated clothing styles for centuries, was the center of the booming fashion industry led by the designers of *haute couture*, or high fashion clothing. Her strong instincts told her that it might also be a good place to continue building her cosmetic empire. One of her sisters took over running the London business and Rubinstein moved to Paris to establish a salon. By the time she arrived in Paris, she had given herself a title and was known as "Madame" Helena Rubinstein. Between 1908 and 1915, Rubinstein focused on building her two European businesses and cultivating friendships in the Parisian arts community. Her third salon did as well as her first two.

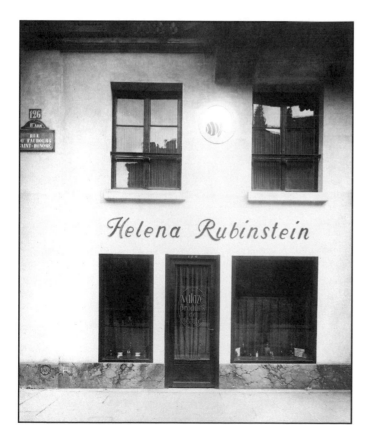

The exterior of Helena Rubinstein's first Paris shop

THE RIVALRY

Prompted by the outbreak of war in Europe in 1914, Rubinstein moved to the United States the following year and opened a salon in New York. It was a good business decision—by the end of the war she had added a wholesale side to her business. Instead of just selling her beauty creams to the women who visited her salons, she produced the creams and lotions in large amounts to sell directly to department stores and other retail outlets. Rubinstein's four shops attracted a growing number of devoted

A Helena Rubinstein outlet counter in a New York City department store

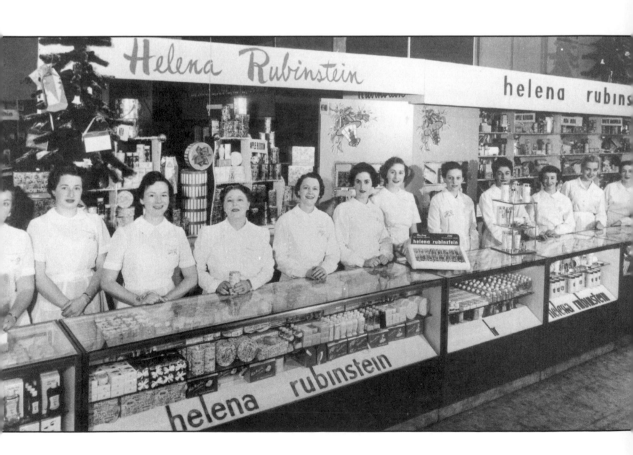

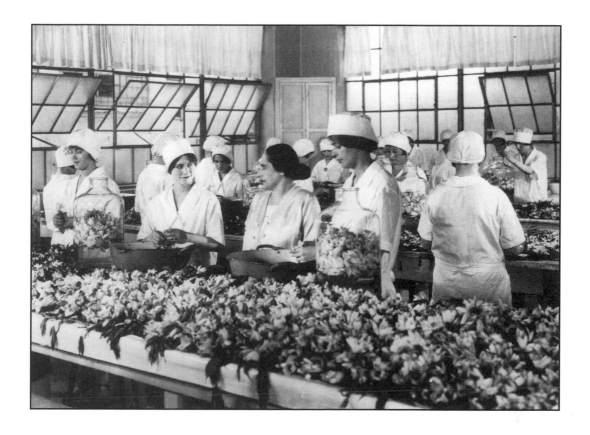

customers, and as more and more women used her products, Helena Rubinstein cosmetics were in great demand. In Australia, she needed to show women how to care for their skin. In London and Paris women had some knowledge of skin care but welcomed her new products. Although Rubinstein was well received elsewhere, in America, one woman, Elizabeth Arden, openly resented Rubinstein's arrival.

Arden also had ambitions about capturing the beauty business in New York City, and she considered it her territory. She thought of Helena Rubinstein as a Polish immigrant who had no place in America.

In order to better handle high-volume product sales, Helena Rubinstein created a manufacturing division in 1917. Here she is shown talking with some of her workers preparing flowers for use in cosmetics.

Rubinstein was terrible at remembering names. Everyone, no matter how long she had known them, ended up with a nickname. Her publicist was "Publicity Woman," and her personal attendant was "The Young Irishman." Elizabeth Arden was "The Other One," and Charles Revson of Revlon became "The Nail Man."

Rubinstein remarried in 1938 to Artchil Gourielli (shown here), an exiled Russian prince. To keep her husband busy, Rubinstein set up the House of Gourielli in New York. Initially selling colognes and knickknacks, in 1953 it was transformed into a men's line called "Gourielli." Other companies had explored the idea of creating cosmetics and toiletry items for men, especially in the early 1930s, but there was a strong perception that men who took too much time on their appearance were effeminate or weak. Rubinstein knew of this perception, but she hoped the success of her women's cosmetics would bolster her men's line. It did not, and the Gourielli men's shop closed in less than a year.

The women did not like each other even though they never met. They even referred to each other as "That woman!" or "That dreadful woman." Once when she was told Elizabeth Arden's horse had bitten off Arden's finger, Rubinstein reportedly responded, "I'm so sorry, is the horse all right?" Whether or not they realized it, they were actually very much alike. Both had strong personalities and ran successful businesses.

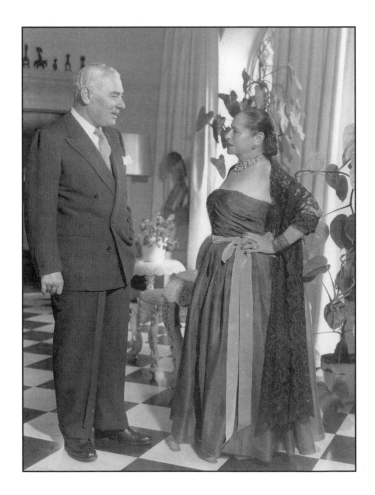

Gillette

Helena Rubinstein's Gourielli line of men's cosmetics folded a year after it debuted. But the failure of one major men's line doesn't mean all early ventures in toiletry products for men were unsuccessful. In 1926, King Camp Gillette said of his first product, the safety razor, "There is no other article for individual use so universally known or widely distributed. . . . I have found it in the most northern town in Norway and in the heart of the Sahara Desert." This distribution was a huge accomplishment for a 25-year-old business that started with just one product.

In 1895, Gillette had what he thought was a great idea for a business. He would make a razor that was sharp enough to give a smooth shave, safe enough for a man to use on himself at home, with conveniently disposable blades. At that time, men who wanted a clean-shaven look had to use an expensive razor blade that needed constant resharpening, or go to the barbershop on a regular basis. Gillette knew the convenience of being able to shave at home, coupled with concerns men had about barbershop hygiene, would make his razor attractive.

Although people were skeptical, Gillette did not give up. His first office was in Boston, and he spent most of his time trying to make his concept of a safety razor a reality. He found a machinist to come up with a model, and even though his idea was simple enough, it took several tries before they found one that worked as Gillette envisioned it. The razor finally went on sale in 1903, and by the end of that year he had sold 51 razors and 168 blades. He considered those sales figures an indication that men were at least interested in an inexpensive safety razor with disposable blades, and he continued to make his razors.

His persistence paid off. By the end of 1904, the Gillette Safety Razor Company had sold almost 91,000 razors and more than 10,000 packages of replacement blades. The company remained focused on making the best possible safety razor blade, and it received a boost in sales when the U.S. government ordered 3.5 million razors and 32 million blades for its servicemen during World War I.

Over the years, the company continued to perfect its product. When King C. Gillette died in 1932 at the age of 77, the company was still improving the single-blade safety razor. In 1972, Gillette introduced a razor with two blades, and in 1993 it created one with three. Disposable razors hit the market in 1976.

One hundred years after the company's birth, Gillette was one of the most recognized names in the world. In addition to razors, it also owned other companies such as Oral B toothbrushes, RightGuard, and Papermate.

TURNING A PROFIT

The Helena Rubinstein Company in England was organized as a foundation to avoid high taxes. The business was a public corporation in the United States. In 1928, Rubinstein sold her interest in the American business to an investment firm called Lehman Brothers. She had always targeted an upscale market and strived to give her products an air of exclusivity, but Lehman Brothers had different plans. They tried to market Helena Rubinstein cosmetics as a cheap variety-store line. Rubinstein was furious and refused to sit by and watch. Shortly after the stock market crash of 1929, she managed to persuade Lehman Brothers to sell her company back to her and took her place once more as president of the American Helena Rubinstein Company. She made a net profit of $6 million in this transaction.

Once she had her company back under her control, Rubinstein continued to produce innovative cosmetics. In 1939, she introduced waterproof mascara, which remained popular into the twenty-first century. She was the first to develop such products as deep cleansers, vitamin enriched skin-care lines, and a face-care line that included pure vitamin C.

A STUDY IN CONTRASTS

Helena Rubinstein became the wealthiest self-made woman in the world. Her New York apartment had 26 rooms and was considered one of the city's most lavish and expensive homes. She kept homes in London, Paris, and Greenwich, Connecticut, as well.

Rubinstein collected elaborate sets of miniature furniture and accessories, and was passionate about art—there were hundreds of pieces throughout her homes and offices, and many on loan to museums. In Paris she had met a wealthy socialite named Misia Sert, who taught her more about selecting artwork. Some of Sert's friends had included the great French artists Henri de Toulouse-Lautrec and Pierre Auguste Renoir. Helena loved having her portrait painted. "Good for publicity, good investment, good for all the empty walls!" she would say. She also loved clothes by designers such as Chanel, Dior, and

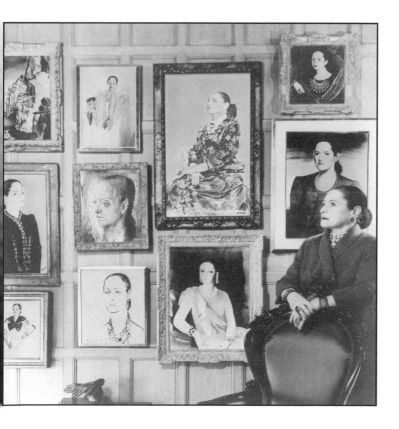

Rubinstein was a passionate art collector; one of her favorite things to acquire was a portrait—of herself. She was both a patron and a friend to many artists, and her likeness was depicted by more than 25 well-known painters, including Graham Sutherland and Salvador Dali. (Sutherland painted the large vertical portrait in the center; Dali produced the one in the upper left corner.)

In 1964, three men rang the doorbell of Rubinstein's New York apartment saying they were delivering flowers. Forcing their way past the butler, they dashed upstairs to the bedroom. Startling Rubinstein in bed, they threatened to kill her if she didn't open her safe. Rubinstein replied, "I'm an old woman, you can kill me. But I'm not going to let you rob me. Now get out." They tied her up, took what money they could find and fled, leaving behind valuable jewelry, antiques, and paintings. Later, Rubinstein said, "Fancy! They ripped my good sheets to tie me up before running out with only a hundred dollars, minus about forty for roses." She was 93 years old.

Balenciaga. But in spite of her collections and love of expensive clothing, Rubinstein did not stray far from her roots. It was not unusual to see her munching on a large Polish sausage while welcoming guests to her sumptuous apartment.

Rubinstein was very generous when it came to helping women. In 1953 she created the Helena Rubinstein Foundation, which offered grants in the areas of the arts, health, education, and community service projects to benefit women and children. "My fortune comes from women," she said, "and should benefit them and their children, to better their quality of life."

LEGACY

Rubinstein died on April 1, 1965, after suffering a stroke the day before. When Elizabeth Arden heard the news she complained, "Why do they have to keep giving her age?" In 1973, the Helena Rubinstein Company was sold to Colgate and in 1988, it was purchased by the French cosmetics company L'Oréal. L'Oréal was considered a leader in the beauty industry, with 49,150 employees and worldwide consolidated sales of almost $16 billion in 2002. L'Oréal's Chief Executive Officer Lindsay Owen-Jones relaunched Helena Rubinstein Cosmetics, targeting women in their 20s and 30s who lived in urban areas. Still considered a luxury cosmetic, the brand was available through selected outlets such as Saks Fifth Avenue and Bergdorf Goodman. Owen-Jones also opened an exclusive yet trendy gallery and spa located in SoHo in New

York City, to showcase the line's newest products and offer luxurious skin treatments.

In 1999, L'Oréal joined with the United Nations Educational Science & Cultural Organization (UNESCO) to establish an award benefitting female researchers in the life sciences. The Helena Rubinstein Awards for Women in Science issued five $20,000 grants to women from all over the world.

Helena Rubinstein believed all women could be beautiful, and she tried to address as many skin-care needs as she could with her cosmetics. Because of her vision, women across many generations were able to see themselves the way she did—as beautiful people.

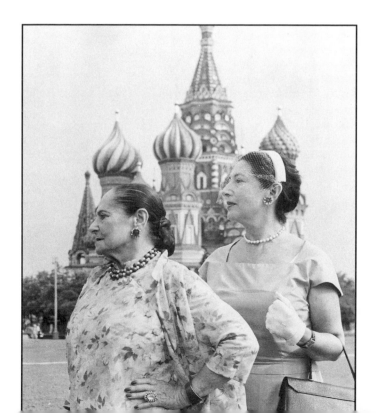

The Helena Rubinstein brand name became associated with glamour, aristocracy, and exclusivity, and Rubinstein's social standing reflected that. When she traveled, she was often greeted with the same reception given to celebrities and political dignitaries. Here, she pauses with her niece, Mala, outside of the Red Palace in Moscow during the 1959 International American Commercial Exhibition.

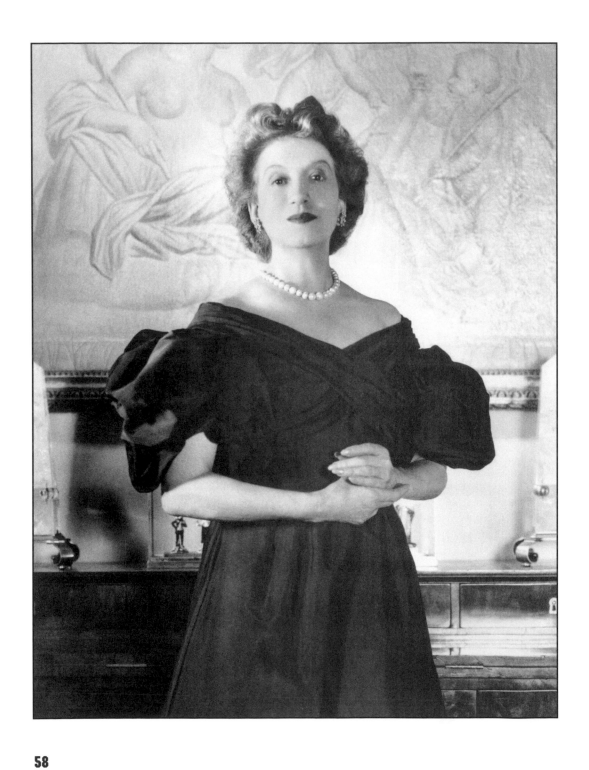

3

ELIZABETH ARDEN

ENTREPRENEUR FOR THE YOUNG AND BEAUTIFUL

Shortly before 4:00 P.M., Elizabeth Arden put away the books she had been reviewing and draped a pink cape over her shoulders. She slid into one of the treatment rooms and waved her hand for an attendant. When the woman finished giving her a facial, Arden grabbed her coat and left the store. Less than an hour later she was back in the office, her skin still radiant from her earlier facial and her left hand bearing evidence of the errand—a wedding ring. She worked until 8:00 P.M., then left to meet her new husband for their wedding supper.

Squeezing her wedding into her work schedule was not really a surprise to those who knew Arden well. She was consumed with building her cosmetics business and spent almost every waking hour looking

A driven, and sometimes ruthless, businesswoman, Elizabeth Arden (1878-1966) helped revolutionize the cosmetics industry in America.

over the books, monitoring her employees, or discussing ideas for new products. Her drive to succeed took her from a farm in Canada to New York City, where she built a multimillion-dollar business that managed to thrive even during the Great Depression.

FLORENCE NIGHTINGALE GRAHAM

Elizabeth Arden was born Florence Nightingale Graham on December 31, 1878, in the small town of Woodbridge, just north of Toronto, Canada. Her parents, William and Susan Graham, had eloped to Canada from Great Britain when Susan's wealthy family opposed their relationship. The couple struggled to find work in Toronto before moving to the town of Woodbridge, where William leased a tenant farm.

By the time Florence was born, the family already included two girls, Lillian and Christine, and one boy, William. Susan wanted to give her third daughter a powerful name, so she called her Florence Nightingale, after her idol, the famous nurse. Susan had one more child, Gladys. This last pregnancy weakened her. She developed tuberculosis and died when Florence was only six years old.

After their mother's death, Florence, or Flo as she was called, took care of the family's horses and went with her father to market. It was on these trips she discovered her knack for sales. The adults who visited her father's stall were amused when she used her baby voice, and they bought more of her father's goods. Neither she nor her father knew how important those early sales experiences would be.

When it was time for her to decide what she would do with her life, Flo chose nursing, like her namesake. She entered nurse's training school, but she did not last long there. "I found I didn't really like looking at sick people," she said. "I want to keep people well, and young, and beautiful."

Although she left school, Flo's experience was not a waste of time. While at the hospital, she met a biochemist who was working on a cream to cure skin blemishes. This gave Flo an idea. Not everyone was blessed with as good a complexion as she was. If a blemish cream were developed for medicinal uses, perhaps it could also be used as a cosmetic by women who did not have perfect skin. Flo decided to attempt to develop a cream on her own that she could sell through the mail. Excited about her idea, Flo spent hours in the family kitchen cooking various substances to make her cream.

THE BIG CITY

After her father put a stop to the experiments and told her to find real employment, Flo Graham took a series of jobs in Toronto. When none of them was to her liking, she announced she was going to New York, where her brother, William, lived. From the minute she arrived, she loved the excitement of the city. Her first job in New York was with a leading manufacturer of pharmaceutical products, E. R. Squibb and Sons. Graham took advantage of her new position to spend time in the company

When Flo began experimenting with making face creams, the smells filling the house became so unbearable that the neighbors told the local clergyman they thought the family was destitute and living on rotten food. After the well-meaning minister paid the family a visit to bring them something to eat, Flo's embarrassed father forced her to stop the experiments.

laboratory asking about substances that might be good for skin care.

In the early 1900s when Graham arrived in New York, there was a growing interest in skin care. All around the city "beauty culturists," who claimed to be able to make skin look younger, opened parlors or salons offering beauty treatments. Graham found a position with Eleanor Adair, one of these beauty culturists. The treatments Adair's salon used involved strapping the customer's jaw closed and massaging creams and oils into the skin. Graham learned quickly, and her strong hands allowed her to give such good facial treatments that customers requested her by name.

After working at the parlor for some time, Graham realized Adair's products were not very good. If she could only develop her own creams, she could do what Adair was doing, and do it even better. In 1909, she met Elizabeth Hubbard, who provided the opportunity Graham had been looking for. Hubbard had skin-care products, but she did not have Graham's "magic hands" to apply them. The two women formed a partnership, planning to open a salon and create a successful business by combining their talents. It didn't take long for their dominant personalities to clash, however, and the partnership fell apart before the business opened. Hubbard moved to a new location, and Graham decided to open the salon on her own.

Graham wanted to name the salon after herself, but "Florence Nightingale" did not seem an appropriate name for a beauty parlor. Besides, the famous nurse had recently died, and Graham did not want her salon associated with mourning. The solution was to change her name. The half-painted name on the window of her salon already said "Elizabeth," so Graham kept it and then brainstormed to find a surname. While reading a volume of poems by Alfred, Lord Tennyson, she found one entitled "Enoch Arden." Arden sounded wonderful when paired with Elizabeth, so she became Elizabeth Arden.

THE FIRST LITTLE STEPS

In 1910, armed with experience from Adair and knowledge of basic formulas from Hubbard, Arden set about preparing for her opening. She borrowed $6,000 from her brother to get started and gave manicures on the side to stay afloat until the business earned money. She created a sumptuous parlor to attract customers. Pink was her favorite color, so she paneled the walls in pink damask. She also purchased a few choice French antiques and an Oriental carpet, and she installed a beautiful Venetian chandelier. She called her creams "Venetian," hoping customers would confuse them with Hubbard's more well-known "Grecian." She also added more fragrance to improve the creams' odor. To attract attention, she installed a bright red front door and hung a brass nameplate on it with her name in script. After hiring a receptionist and two treatment women, Elizabeth Arden opened her salon for business.

damask: a heavy fabric of cotton, silk, linen, or wool woven with elaborate patterns

Arden had an extra rear parlor in her salon and, rather than leave it empty, she rented it to Jessica and Clara Ogilvie, sisters who gave hair and scalp treatments that Arden knew would be a wonderful addition to her salon. She was so confident about her business's future she announced to the sisters, "You're so very fortunate. Just think—you'll be here to watch me take my first little steps."

ADDING A LITTLE COLOR

Just as she knew it would, Arden's business made money, and she repaid her brother's loan in just six

The familiar facade of Elizabeth Arden's 5th Avenue Salon in New York. The red door of the salon became a trademark for Arden and was so well recognized that she named a perfume after it. Today, the Red Door fragrance is one of the company's most popular scents.

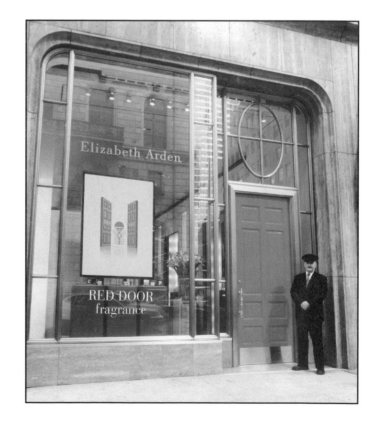

months. She spent the remaining profits on making improvements in her salon and her formulas. "You've got to spend a little money to make a little money," she said. She arrived early to clean the salon and stayed late to work on her formulas in the laboratory. Soon the business became her life.

In 1912, *Vogue* magazine announced that a "discreet application of a little paint would enhance a lady's appearance." This small statement opened the door for Arden to develop rouges and tinted powders, and she discovered she had a talent for blending colors to create shades appealing to her customers. When beauty culturists first started experimenting with color, the cheek rouges they worked with were in very bright shades. If not properly blended, they looked garish and ridiculous. Arden practiced applying the colors on her employees until she developed a way of using rouge that looked natural.

The amazing growth of her business convinced Arden it was time to expand. In 1914, she got her first bank loan and opened a branch of her salon in Washington, D.C. As the owner of two salons, Arden needed to improve her knowledge of cosmetics, and she realized the place to do so was Paris. She arrived in France the same month that World War I broke out.

STUDYING HER CRAFT IN PARIS

Undeterred by the fact that Europe was at war, Arden visited many salons to experience and observe their treatment methods. She knew immediately

Arden's devotion to her business never wavered. Obsessed with the details of running her company, she had only one passion outside of it—her prizewinning racehorses. One of these, Jet Pilot, was the 1947 Kentucky Derby winner, and Arden was featured on the cover of *Time* magazine for her success in racing. The magazine called her "a queen [ruling] the sport of kings."

One of the main reasons Arden decided to go to Paris to improve her knowledge of cosmetics was, essentially, to spy on Madame Helena Rubinstein. Rubinstein was already well established in Europe, and had done much to mainstream cosmetic use there.

the French were far ahead of Americans in the beauty business. Arden was stunned to find women in Paris wearing eye shadow and mascara, applied so subtly it took her a while to figure out what they were wearing. She had thought only "loose" women and actresses wore such makeup, but the French women looked elegant. She immediately bought samples of everything she found. Her trip to Paris had been exactly the education she hoped it would be, and she was eager to begin experimenting in her laboratory. She also wanted to begin work on a perfume line. Filled with excitement, Arden returned home.

EXPANDING THE LINE

Arden soon realized her plans to add colors and fragrances and to expand her skin-care line were far beyond the scope of her little lab. At a company called Stillwell and Gladding she found a chemist, A. Fabian Swanson, who agreed to help. The chemist analyzed her products and created new ones based on the specifications she provided. In particular, Arden wanted her creams to have the texture of whipped cream instead of the hard and oily texture of many on the market.

Swanson soon developed the light, fluffy product Arden had envisioned; she named it Venetian Cream Amoretta. It felt velvety smooth on the skin and could be used as both a skin softener and base for powder. Thrilled with the results, Arden asked Swanson to create a gentle lotion to replace the strong, alcohol-based ones women were using to

After developing Venetian Cream Amoretta, A. Fabian Swanson created a skin lotion for Arden, which she named "Ardena Skin Tonic." This marked the first time a specific cosmetic was named for its maker.

tone their skin after cleansing. Swanson created this and many more exclusive products for Arden, including a pore cream for blackheads, an oil to combat wrinkles, and a cream to keep the neck and bust firm.

Arden was determined to lead the way with color cosmetics, and soon, in addition to her skin-care items, she had a full line of rouges and tinted face powders, which she urged her customers to try. At first they resisted because wearing color cosmetics still carried some stigma, but eventually women began to feel they were on the leading edge of a new trend and wore more and more of Arden's color cosmetics.

EXPANDING IN EUROPE

Elizabeth Arden was a success. She was earning money, had a good reputation, and had expanded her headquarters, but she was lonely. Aside from the people with whom she worked, she had almost no friends. On May 8, 1915, she received a call from Tommy Lewis. Lewis was a banker who had given Arden her first loan. They had met again and become close when she was sailing home from Europe on the *Lusitania*. After returning to America, however, Arden told Lewis she needed to focus on her business, and the two parted ways. When Lewis called her that May, he had shocking news: a German submarine had sunk the British ocean liner they had traveled on. One thousand people, including 114 Americans, died. The two met to talk about the tragedy and soon rekindled their romantic

Arden led the way in more than just product innovations. In 1920, she began a promotion encouraging women to write to her describing their skin problems. She would answer, recommending specific Arden products to help their conditions. This eventually led to the creation of company newsletters, a practice that became an industry standard.

relationship. When he proposed marriage, she accepted.

Not long after their quiet wedding, Lewis left to fight in World War I. When he returned, he took over Arden's company books. He and Arden went on a delayed honeymoon to Europe, where they toured England to explore the possibility of opening a salon. Also on the trip to Europe was Arden's youngest sister, Gladys Baraba. She had come along in order to visit France and investigate the cosmetics market there. While Arden and Lewis were

Arden and husband Tommy Lewis on their wedding day in 1915

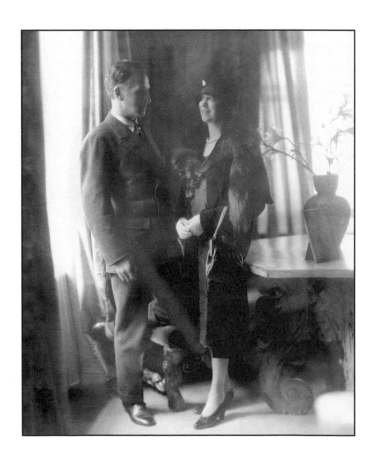

negotiating with the British, Baraba traveled to Paris to introduce the Arden products. She convinced Raul Mayer, head of the French store Galeries Lafayette, to let her open a stall in his store to sell Arden cosmetics. She did so well she was able to train an assistant to take over. Eventually, she convinced Arden to open a factory in France and hire chemists to produce Elizabeth Arden products and develop new ones designed to appeal to European women.

With the Paris business growing and England showing promise, Lewis had an idea to increase profits in the United States. He believed it was time to be selective about the outlets that carried the Arden products. In 1920, he made Arden products available only in New York stores located along prestigious Fifth Avenue. He continued this selective marketing in other cities across the country. The company would focus its sales on the wealthy women who associated exclusivity and price with quality. The strategy paid off, and in spite of the fact that Arden now only targeted the top three percent of the female population in America, the company grossed more than $2 million in domestic wholesale sales in 1925. Elizabeth boasted, "There are only three American names that are known in every corner of the globe. Singer Sewing Machines, Coca-Cola, and Elizabeth Arden."

THAT WOMAN!

Despite their successful business, Arden and Lewis had problems in their marriage, and they divorced in

Elizabeth's youngest sister, Gladys, stayed in France after opening the Arden salons, and eventually married a minor nobleman, Henri de Maublanc. During the German occupation in World War II, Gladys was caught helping Allied pilots escape German territory and was imprisoned in the Ravensbrück concentration camp until the summer of 1944. After being freed and regaining her strength, Gladys resumed her position as head of Elizabeth Arden's French division.

Arden insisted all her salesmen be over six feet tall—it gave her the feeling that she was dainty.

1934. Arden had purchased property in Maine she called Maine Chance, but her sadness over the divorce and the death of her good friend and neighbor Bessie Marbury lessened her enjoyment of the property. In 1934, she converted it into a luxurious health spa where women came for healthy food, skin-care treatments, and exercise (it was one of the first health spas to offer an exercise class). Arden also recorded her exercise routines and sold the records.

The cosmetics industry in the early years was extremely competitive. The owners of the top companies were aware of each other's every move, and

Maine Chance. It was originally built as a vacation home, but Arden later turned it into a luxury spa where women would pay as much as $500 a week (at the height of the Great Depression) to eat very little and exercise a lot in an attempt to lose weight.

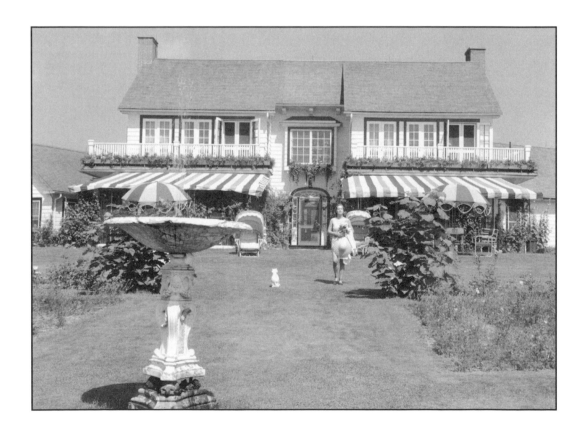

when Helena Rubinstein opened her New York salon, Arden decided she also needed new quarters. She and Rubinstein became serious competitors, referring to each other as "that woman," waging war with their ads, and hiring each other's staff. Rubinstein hired Tommy Lewis, Arden's ex-husband, to work for her, and Arden, to retaliate, hired Harry Johnson, who at that time worked for Rubinstein. Johnson brought 11 of Rubinstein's employees with him when he came to Arden. Both women even entered the men's skin-care market at around the same time, and, ironically, both married exiled princes after divorcing their first husbands!

Like her rival Helena Rubinstein, Elizabeth Arden also married an exiled Russian prince. Unlike Rubinstein's marriage, however, Arden's union was not a blissful one. Michael Evanloff and Elizabeth Arden married in 1942, began fighting on their honeymoon, and divorced a year later.

An Innovative Leader

Arden had a difficult time filling Lewis's role in the company after their divorce. She lost $500,000 in the first two years after he left. Ultimately, she weathered the crisis, recovered financially, and continued to lead the industry with her innovations.

During the Great Depression, a time when many businesses were forced to cut back or even close their doors, Elizabeth Arden continued to spend money. Shortly after the stock market crashed in 1929, she bought an office building and a penthouse in New York. She also opened several salons during the 1930s. Arden loved to drop in on her stores unexpectedly, saying, "It keeps everybody on their toes, dear." Around this time Arden also developed the Youth Mask—a mask made from papier-mâché and insulated with foil. The mask was designed to replenish the cells in a woman's face by applying small

In 1932, Elizabeth Arden introduced a palette of lipstick shades in a kit whose colors were designed to match a woman's outfits. Arden followed this by offering mascara, and then more powders and rouges, in ensemble shades. Until then, women bought a few shades of makeup that complimented their own skin and hair tones. Now they could match their colors to their clothing. This ad suggests that women love the "harmony between costume colors and lipstick shades" that Elizabeth Arden products created.

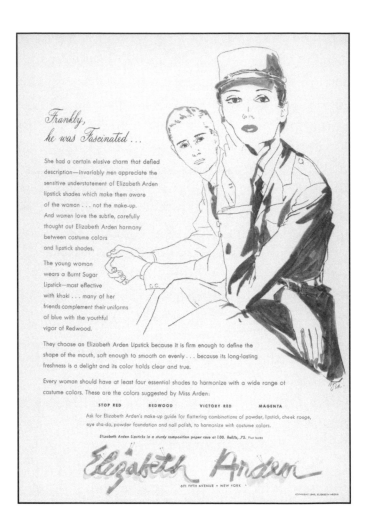

amounts of electric currents to it. Arden's chemist, Swanson, also developed the Eight Hour Cream, which became one of the company's most popular products. The cream worked so well on skin abrasions and burns that even children's hospitals used it. In 1936, Arden added hairdressing departments to her salons. She also made a foray into the fragrance market that yielded a number of popular scents. One perfume, called Blue Grass, was named in honor of Arden's passion for horseracing. Critics said with a name like that, it would never sell. She proved them wrong, and Blue Grass went on to become the top-selling fragrance of that time.

LEGACY

By the time she died in October 1966, Elizabeth Arden had been given many prestigious honors and awards. She received an honorary Doctorate of Law from Syracuse University for "enriching American standards." The Woodbridge, Canada, farm where she was born and grew up was made into a park called Dalziel Pioneer Park. She was one of the

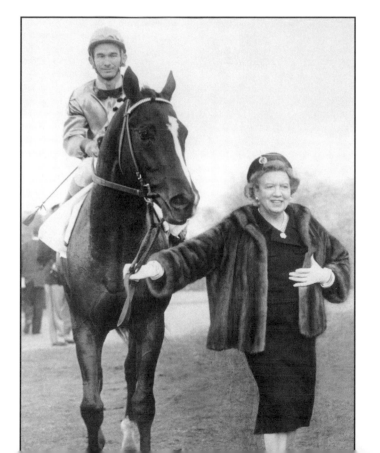

Arden treated her racehorses very well. The stable was decorated in pink and white, with plants hanging over the stalls and soothing music playing. The horses wore perfume, their blankets were cashmere, and once, when one horse was ill, Arden called the Mayo Clinic for a diagnosis. Arden also had $10-a-jar Eight Hour Cream rubbed on their bruises instead of petroleum jelly and had them rubbed down with Ardena skin lotion. Even after one horse, Jewel's Reward (left), bit off the tip of her finger, Arden still called him "her darling."

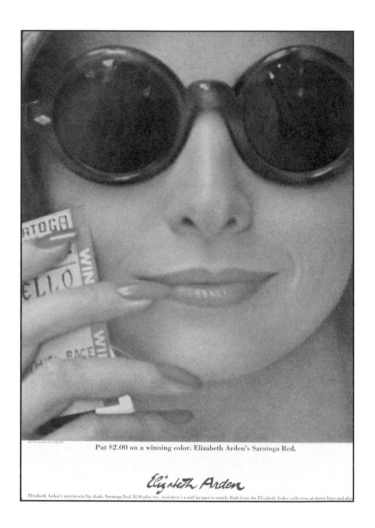

Put $2.00 on a winning color. Elizabeth Arden's Saratoga Red.

Elizabeth Arden

Elizabeth Arden's sure-to-win lip shade, Saratoga Red, $2.00 plus tax. And there's a nail lacquer to match. Both from the Elizabeth Arden collection at stores here and also

Arden named many of her scents and colors after horse-related themes. This 1963 ad is for Saratoga Red lipstick and nail enamel, which were named after the famous Saratoga racetrack in New York.

Arden became an American citizen when she married Tommy Lewis in 1915.

judges of the Miss America Pageant in 1952. Arden was the first American citizen to receive the Golden Cup of the Comité du Bon Gout Français for the creation of her French perfume Mémoire Chérie. Her close friendship with First Lady Mamie Eisenhower earned her the unofficial title of "beauty maker to the Republican administration."

Arden's interests went beyond skin care, and she also helped women in other areas of their lives. She introduced *haute couture*, or high fashion, to her salons, first by hiring people to copy French clothing designs, then by hiring her own designers. Just before World War II, when America's involvement in the conflict seemed inevitable, she designed courses for women to help prepare them for their new wartime roles. Her courses helped women select clothing for a work environment and also gave information about exercise, diet, makeup, and grooming for hair and nails.

Following Arden's death, her general manager, Carl Gardiner, was appointed president of the Elizabeth Arden Company. In 1971, the company was sold to pharmaceutical manufacturer Eli Lilly and Company, and sold again in 1986 to Faberge. Unilever purchased Faberge and Elizabeth Arden in 1989. In January 2001, a small fragrance company called FFI Fragrances bought Arden and announced it would change its company name to Elizabeth Arden, Inc.

Despite all the changes, the Elizabeth Arden label continued to be recognized as a symbol of quality, representing a company that offered such products as a long-wearing, breath-freshening lipstick and Custom Color Foundation that helped women match their foundation to their skin color and type.

Even after more than 90 years, the Elizabeth Arden Company continues to appeal to customers who, like the company's founder, are confident, determined women pursuing their own goals and dreams.

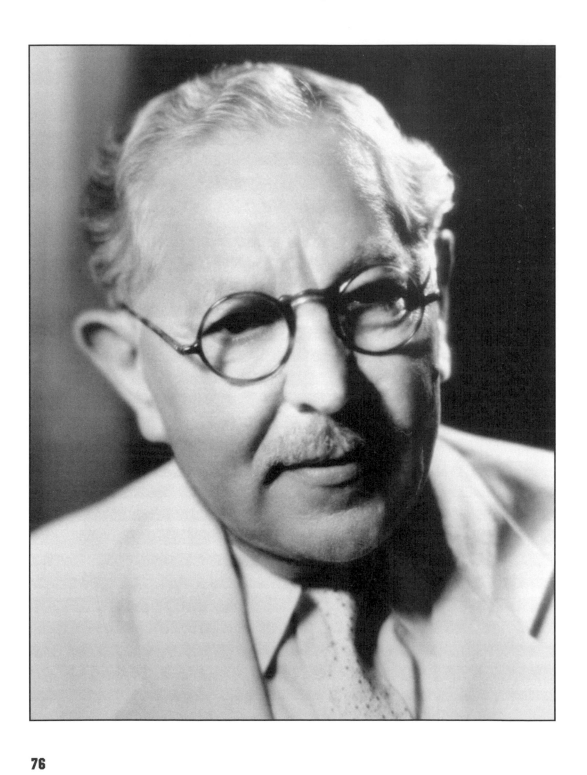

4

MAX FACTOR

MAKEUP ARTIST
TO THE STARS

In the privacy of his bedroom, Max Faktor carefully applied makeup to his face. He chose a shade that made him look tired and sickly. It was a long shot, but if his employer at the Russian court thought he was sick enough to need rest, he might send him to Carlsbad to get well. It was 1904, and for as long as Faktor could remember, members of the Russian royal family had gone to that resort to recover from illnesses.

There was a knock at his door. He rose and moved to answer. This had to work. Just minutes later, Faktor reentered his room and shut the door behind him. Only then did he smile. Brilliant! His trick had succeeded and he was going to Carlsbad to recover from his "illness." Now he, Lizzie, and their

Max Factor Sr. (1872-1938) brought movie-star glamour to the everyday lives of women.

children could escape Russia and flee to America. He patted his makeup case—his ticket to freedom.

POLISH ROOTS

Max Faktor was born in Lodz, Poland, sometime in the 1870s. His year of birth is sometimes given as 1872, 1874, or 1877; even Max himself did not know the actual date. (According to his biographer, Fred E. Basten, 1872 seems to be the most plausible year.) His Jewish parents, Abraham and Cecilia Tandowsky Faktor, had 10 children. The Faktors did not have enough money to send their children to formal schools; instead, they apprenticed them to local merchants to learn trades. Max was sent to assist a dentist-apothecary when he was eight years old. Later he was apprenticed to a wig maker, where he learned how to tie human hair onto a foundation made of silk. His skill as a fledgling wig maker earned him a position with the Imperial Russian Grand Opera.

During Max's youth, much of the eastern part of Poland was under Russian control, and the law required that all young men serve in the Russian army when they turned 18. Max hoped to be allowed to work in military dramatics during his time in the army, but he was chosen for the Hospital Corps. Instead of helping stage performances, he learned how to bleed patients with leeches.

MAX AND LIZZIE

In 1894, Faktor completed his time in the army and opened a small shop in R'azan, a suburb of Moscow.

apothecary: a person who prepares and sells drugs and other medicines; a pharmacist

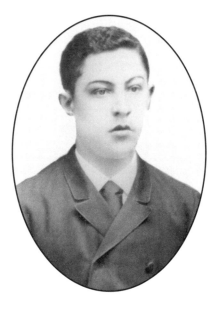

Max at about the age of 16. When this picture was taken he was working with the Imperial Russian Grand Opera as a wigmaker.

He sold face creams, rouges, fragrances, and wigs—all products he made himself. He might have expected to live out the rest of his life as a simple merchant, but his small shop attracted people in high places and led him on a different path. According to legend, some traveling performers shopped at his store, and when the Russian nobility saw their performances, they also saw Faktor's makeup and wigs. Before long, members of Tsar Nicholas II's royal court became his customers, and eventually he was made cosmetic consultant to the royal family. This position, though prestigious, cost Faktor his

Faktor's first shop in R'azan. He is standing on the far right in the doorway.

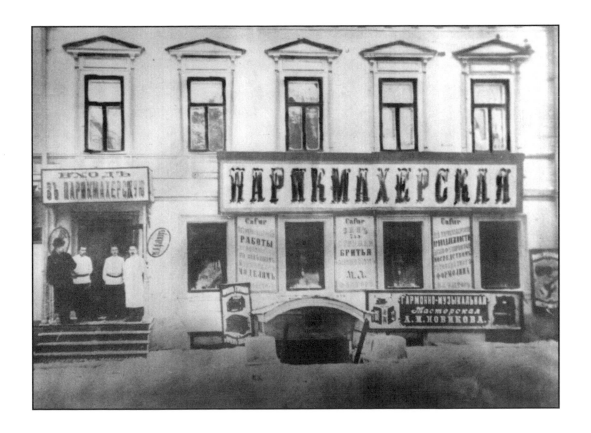

freedom. He was under constant guard and was expected to be available to tend to the royal family's needs at all times.

Faktor had everything he could possibly want, but he was not content. His thoughts were on a young lady he had met when he first opened his shop. Esther Rosa, who Faktor called Lizzie, had come to R'azan to buy perfume. She seemed to like him as much as he liked her, because after that first visit she came once each week.

When Faktor was appointed cosmetician to the tsar's family, he was allowed only one day off per week, yet he and Lizzie continued to see each other secretly. They even managed to marry and have three children: Freda, Cecilia, and Davis. They kept their secret for almost nine years! But as the children grew up, Faktor grew more and more unhappy with his situation. He was earning a lot of money, but he could only see his wife and children once every week, and he wanted a normal life. He decided to leave the royal court, but knew if he did that he would also have to leave Russia.

A New Life in a New World

The decision to leave Russia was not a difficult one for Max and Lizzie. Max already had a brother and an uncle who had moved to the city of St. Louis in the United States, and it seemed a logical place for Faktor to move his family. When his brother wrote to tell him of the magnificent 1904 World's Fair, where Faktor could display his wigs and perfumes, he started to make plans to leave. Once Faktor had fooled his employers into letting him leave the palace, he, Lizzie, and the children sneaked across the countryside until they reached the nearest seaport. On February 13, 1904, they left for America on the ship *Molka III*.

Faktor's first order of business was to prepare for the World's Fair. He met a man while on board the *Molka III* who became his partner and helped him secure a small space to show his goods. (He also got a new name: during his processing on Ellis Island, the name Faktor was "Americanized" to Factor.)

The World's Fair ran for seven months and would have been a wonderful way to launch Factor into business in America—except that when the fair ended his partner disappeared and took Factor's money and all his merchandise. He and Lizzie were left with nothing. Factor did not have time to wallow in despair; he needed to find a way to earn a living for his wife and three children. With help from his brother and uncle, he opened a barbershop and began cutting hair. He and his family lived in an apartment above the shop.

Gradually, he began to earn enough money to pay back his relatives and put a little away as savings. Soon, the Factors welcomed a new baby boy, Frank (later Max Jr.), to the family. Just when it seemed they had managed to overcome their initial setback, Lizzie died suddenly from a brain hemorrhage. Not only was Lizzie's death a huge blow to Max, but he also realized that after living without their father for so long, his children desperately needed the stability of a two-parent home. He wrote to a family friend

Many immigrants to the United States, especially those who came between 1880 and 1920, "Americanized" their names to blend in better with society. For example, a German name like "Schmidt" might become "Smith."

in Russia asking permission to marry one of the friend's daughters.

Huma, his new wife, was much younger than Max, and even after their son, Louis, was born, it was clear the relationship would not work. They divorced. The trauma of losing two wives in so short a time faded, however, when he fell in love with his neighbor, Jennie Cook. The children also loved her, and the couple married on January 21, 1908.

MOVIES AND MAKEUP

With his home life in order, Max Factor turned his attention to the future. Even though his barber-shop was doing well in 1908, his heart was really not in the business. He had been listening with interest to stories about the movie industry growing

The Factor family in about 1917. Back row (left to right): Max Jr., Cecilia, Freda; front row (left to right): Davis, Jennie holding baby Sydney, Louis, Max Sr.

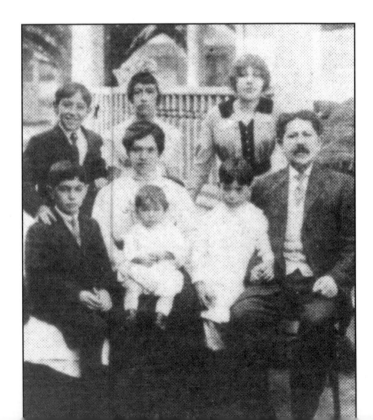

in California. He thought he might be able to make a decent living selling wigs and cosmetics to the people working on the motion pictures.

On October 11, 1908, Factor moved his family to Los Angeles. The move was a smart one for Factor because, while industry growth was slow at first, by the end of 1911, 154 film companies were making films in Los Angeles or in a suburb near it called Hollywood. By then Factor was creating and selling a small line of cosmetics: face powder, cleansing cream, and lip rouge. He had become the West Coast distributor for two companies, Leichtner and Minor, that manufactured stick greasepaint used by theater performers as well as the new movie actors. When Factor sold his makeup, he showed his customers how to apply the products so they would look their best on the stage or the screen. Word about Factor's skill gradually spread throughout the growing Los Angeles community, and the stars came to him for tips on makeup application as well as to buy his goods. In the early days, the movie studios did not have makeup departments, and actors generally had to figure out how to apply it on their own. In 1917, this began to change with Paramount's film *Joan the Woman*, starring Geraldine Farrar. The script took makeup concerns into consideration, and Factor was hired to supervise the cast's makeup.

MAX FACTOR BECOMES AN INNOVATOR

Factor was a huge fan of the movies, and he knew screen actors were having trouble with the greasepaint originally created for stage performers. He

greasepaint: a type of theatrical makeup, usually made by combining a preparation of grease with colors

When the motion-picture industry began, the only foundation for the new movie actors was the same greasepaint originally designed for stage actors. It came in stick form and had to be applied at least one-eighth of an inch thick and then powdered. When it dried, it cracked and created fine lines on the actors' faces. In the theater, this had not been a huge problem because the audience sat far away from the actors. On film, however, especially during closeups, the little lines were visible, and actors had to remain almost expressionless to avoid the cracks.

began experimenting in his small lab to find a foundation the screen actors could use. In June 1914, he came up with greasepaint in cream form. It was thinner and more flexible than the old stick form of greasepaint. When applied, it allowed the actors to use a full range of facial expressions. For comedians such as Charlie Chaplin and Roscoe "Fatty" Arbuckle, whose facial expressions were a crucial part of their performances, the cream greasepaint was a dream come true. Movie actors began coming to Factor's store to buy the new makeup.

Cream greasepaint was the first of many innovative products Factor and his sons would develop to

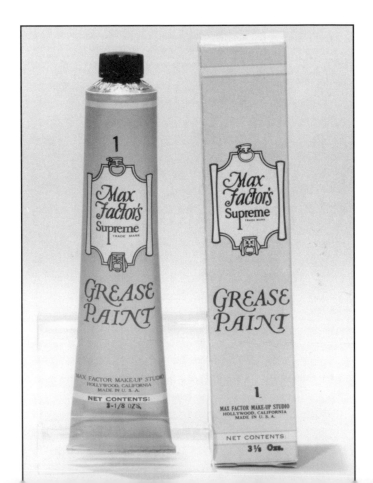

Max Factor's greasepaint in tube form. The product came in 31 shades, including White, Very Light Pink, Sunburn, Dark Brown, and Black. Each shade had its own number.

meet the needs of the movie industry. When the handsome leading man Rudolph Valentino asked Factor to create a shade of makeup that complemented his dark olive skin, Factor developed one that worked well with the actor's skin tones and improved Valentino's appearance on film.

Factor's interest in different makeup shades led to the development of his "Color Harmony" principles in 1918. After working with Valentino and other actors, he learned that certain combinations of hair, skin, and eye color looked best when paired with makeup colors that harmonized with them. This knowledge led to more predictable makeup effects on screen.

Factor believed these principles would also work for women outside the movie industry, and he made a mental note to pursue marketing them to the public in the future. In 1918, a few women were experimenting with makeup, but putting color on the face was still considered somewhat improper. In the 1920s, Factor followed his earlier instincts and marketed a makeup specifically for everyday use. Society Make-Up, as he called it, allowed women outside the movie industry to try the cosmetics they knew were made by the same company that helped their favorite movie stars look beautiful.

A GROWING BUSINESS

As Factor became known in Los Angeles, his business grew. In the first part of the 1920s, he moved his shop to the heart of the film district: the prestigious Pantages Theater building on South Hill

One busy day, Factor arrived at a studio in the morning to put a black eye on actor Ben Turpin, then dashed off to another studio. When Factor returned later in the day to reapply Turpin's black eye, he painted the wrong eye. The mistake was not caught in the editing, and when Factor viewed the film for the first time and saw the actor's black eye switch from one side to the other he was terribly embarrassed. The director loved it and kept it in the film, calling it "great shtick."

Street in downtown Los Angeles. In 1928, Factor moved the shop again, this time to Hollywood, where, as word spread about his services, famous movie stars clamored for his cosmetics.

When Factor introduced greasepaint in tubes, his brand outsold both greasepaint companies he had previously represented. Sold as the world's first "sanitary" greasepaint (Factor felt that the stick form was unhygienic), it became the best-selling brand on the market.

Factor continued to develop new products. As lighting and film changed, so did makeup. The

The "Max Factor House of Make-Up" on South Hill Street in downtown Los Angeles around 1920

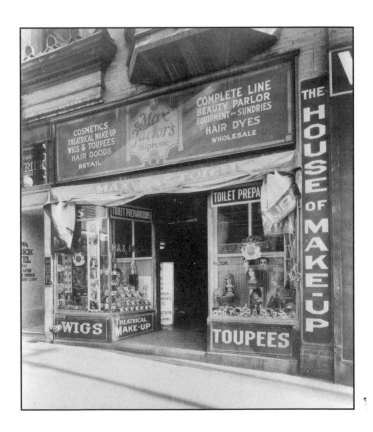

lights used on the movie set of *The Jazz Singer* (1927) were hotter than those on previous sets, and the film itself was more sensitive. Makeup needed to be thinner and more transparent than before.

When color film was introduced, makeup required an even more dramatic change. With black-and-white film, the goal was to make the skin appear smooth and unblemished. With color, the old greasepaint reflected colors from the scenery around the actors. Their faces looked red or green or blue depending on their surroundings. Actors were actually afraid to make films in Technicolor, thinking their bizarre skin tones in this medium would ruin their careers.

In response, Max and his son Frank came up with "Pan-Cake" makeup, which was used for the first time in 1937 on the cast members of the film *Vogues of 1938*. This makeup had a nonreflective transparent matte finish and came in a wide range of Color Harmony tints. It received rave reviews and became the standard for all Technicolor films. Movie stars began requesting "Pan-Cake" for personal use, and Factor eventually released it to the public. It became, according to Factor biographer Fred E. Basten, the "fastest and largest selling single makeup item in the history of cosmetics."

MARKETING MAX FACTOR

In 1928, after Factor's Society Make-Up for the general public received wider distribution, a company called Sales Builders, Inc., was given an exclusive contract to handle all advertising,

The term "makeup" had traditionally been used when referring to paints and theatrical products, and had negative connotations in the early years of the twentieth century. In the 1920s, Factor began calling all his cosmetic products makeup. His name was so associated with glamour that the term took on a favorable, rather than unfavorable, meaning, and all his competitors were forced to use it.

Maybelline

Women in ancient Greece brushed incense on their eyelashes and eyebrows to make them appear darker; a Sanskrit text about love and romance included a recipe for a product that women could apply to their eyelashes as a beauty enhancer. It wasn't until the early part of the twentieth century, however, that mascara was widely accepted as a household cosmetic. Around the time Max Factor was beginning to build his reputation as a makeup artist to Hollywood stars, T. L. Williams was launching his new line of eye makeup.

In about 1913, Williams was watching his older sister, Mabel, apply a concoction of petroleum jelly and coal dust to her eyelashes. Deciding that other women might be interested in his sister's secret trick, Williams formed his company in 1915 and called it Maybelline in her honor.

The company's first product was Cake Mascara. Unlike today's mascara, this product came in the form of a tiny cake. The user would wet a small brush and rub it on the cake until enough of the mascara had collected, and then apply it to her eyelashes. Williams advertised and sold his Cake Mascara by mail. Eyebrow pencils followed, and then a limited number of eye-shadow colors.

In spite of mascara's initial reputation as being a makeup item worn by "racy" girls, Mabel's desire for it seemed to be universal among American women, and they began asking for mascara at their local drugstores. It was not offered in stores, however, until the 1930s, when 10-cent packages of Maybelline Mascara went on sale around the country.

Two products, Ultra Lash Mascara and Great Lash Mascara, put the company on top of the mascara market. Ultra Lash was introduced in the early 1960s and was one of the first "automatic" mascaras—mascara applied directly to the brush in the tube. Great Lash, introduced in 1971, was a water-based mascara with a carefully guarded secret formula. According to the Maybelline company, a Great Lash mascara is sold once every 1.5 seconds.

From eye makeup, Maybelline branched out into other cosmetics categories, including face powders and lip and nail colors. One of the company's most successful ventures was its Express Finish Fast-Dry Nail Enamel introduced in 1997. It was billed as an enamel that "goes from wet to set in one minute." Express Finish nail enamel went on to become the number-one-selling nail polish on the market.

In 1996, Maybelline was sold to L'Oréal USA, Inc., a company known for its emphasis on research and development. In 2003, Maybelline continued to be one of the leading color cosmetic companies in the world.

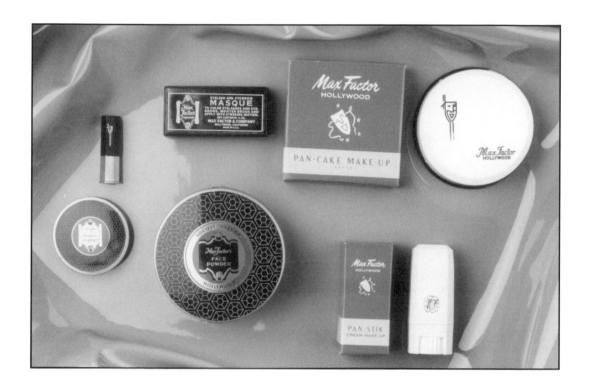

distribution, and sales of Max Factor's products throughout the United States. It came up with a number of ways to catapult Max Factor onto the national market, such as presenting testimonials from famous actresses and using drugstores as outlets for his makeup.

The top three sales executives at Sales Builders actually posed as clerks and worked behind the counters of various drugstores so they could see firsthand how women shopped for cosmetics. They learned women tended to buy one brand of face powder, another of rouge, and another of lipstick. Their goal was to persuade women to purchase all three items from Factor. With this in mind, Factor

Society Make-Up and Pan-Cake Make-Up. Although Society Make-Up was created for everyday wear, Pan-Cake Make-Up was meant to be used by performers in Technicolor movies. After actresses started stealing cases of it from movie sets to give to their friends, however, Factor decided to make it available to the public as well.

developed a "Color Harmony Prescription Make-Up Chart" that helped women identify which Max Factor powder, rouge, and lipstick shades complemented each other and worked best with their own complexion and eye coloring.

WIGS AND HAIRPIECES

While Factor was building a successful cosmetics business, he continued to make wigs. When Factor arrived in Hollywood, the wigs available for actors were made out of everything from straw to tobacco leaves, and on screen they looked obviously fake.

An employee (or "mixer") examines samples of hair in the processing room of the Max Factor wig department. Mixers would blend individual strands of different colored hair together until the wig's shade was exactly right.

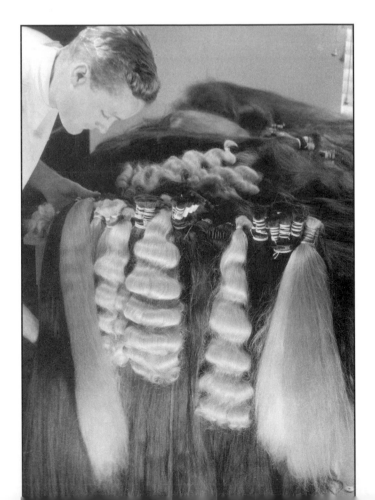

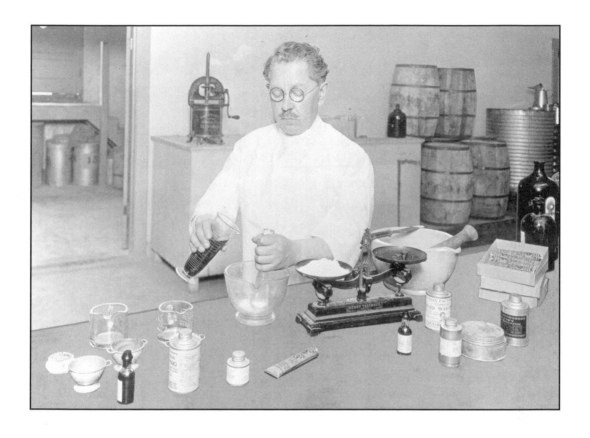

Factor's wigs were extremely realistic because he used only pure virgin hair (hair that had never been dyed or chemically altered by perms). He knew they would look much better on film than the wigs then being used. Another reason he thought movie producers might be interested in his wigs was that the female stars sometimes required as many as six different hairstyles during one day of shooting. Each hairstyle change meant time spent with a stylist and sitting under a dryer. Factor thought it would be more economical and less time-consuming for both male and female stars to wear wigs or hairpieces.

Max Factor Sr. at work in the laboratory in the basement of his shop

Since Cecil B. DeMille had rented, not bought, the hair-pieces for *The Squaw Man*, Factor had his sons cast as extras so they could scramble around after the scenes and collect all the wigs, making sure none were lost.

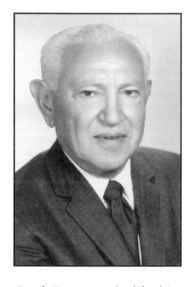

Frank Factor worked for his father since he was a small child. It was fitting that after his father's death, he would not only adopt his father's name, becoming Max Factor Jr., but also take over the business as well.

When Factor approached director Cecil B. DeMille to try his wigs in the movie *The Squaw Man* (1914), DeMille agreed to rent them. The director was delighted with the natural hair wigs and hair-pieces, and after that almost no one used imitation wigs in movies. Max Factor's hair department stayed busy until it closed in 1973, when less expensive, over-the-counter synthetic wigs had become available.

FACTOR PASSES THE BATON

Max Factor died on August 30, 1938, but his name was so tied to his company that publicity director Bill Hardwick suggested Factor's son Frank, who had worked most closely with his father in the lab, should take the name Max Factor Jr.

Max Factor Jr. continued his father's tradition of creating innovative products to meet the needs of the film industry. He developed a cream makeup called "Pan-Stik" that was nongreasy and nonoily as well as "fool proof." Users just needed to remove the cap, twist the base until the makeup appeared, swipe it on the face, and blend it. During World War II, the company adapted experimental body paint to produce a camouflage makeup for the Marine Corps. Factor also developed a new makeup for actors on black-and-white television and then for color television. The company expanded both nationally and overseas and in 1950 introduced a new makeup line called "World of Beauty." In 1961, the company bought Parfums Corday, Inc., and focused on the fragrance market.

LEGACY

Max Factor & Co. had always been a family company. At the end of the 1960s, many of the first generation of family members left to pursue their own interests, and the grandsons stepped in and ran the company until 1976. Beginning in the early 1970s, a series of changes occurred with Max Factor & Co., Inc. The company merged with Norton Simon, Inc., in 1973, and in 1983, Norton Simon was taken over by Esmark, which then merged with Beatrice Companies. With that merger, Max Factor & Co. became a part of International Playtex Division, a company known for making women's undergarments and personal hygiene items. In 1986, Max Factor & Co. was sold to Ron Perelman, owner of Revlon, and then, in 1991, the company was taken over by Procter & Gamble. Throughout all the turmoil of takeovers, acquisitions, and changes, Max Factor & Co. retained its reputation as an innovative company, pioneering foundations and color cosmetics designed to meet the needs of the growing movie and television industry.

Max Factor Sr. began his career serving members of the Russian elite who could afford anything and everything they wanted. He ended his life bringing glamour into the daily lives of ordinary American women.

"No makeup is good makeup, unless the other fellow doesn't know you have it on."
—Max Factor Sr.

93

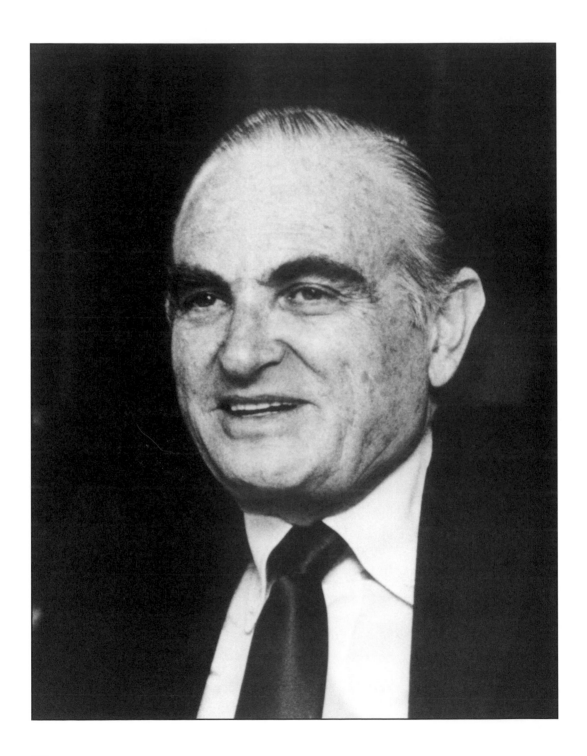

5

CHARLES REVSON

BEGINNING WITH NAILS

The hotel conference room was filled with cosmetics salespeople. They had traveled from all over the country to Asbury Park, New Jersey, to attend this sales meeting and hear Charles Revson, the dynamic owner of Revlon Cosmetics, speak. As they waited, they noticed some activity near the podium, and the room grew quiet. Waiters and waitresses began crisscrossing the room, removing all the place settings and tablecloths from the tables! The salespeople wondered if this was a new sales gimmick.

Once new tablecloths were brought out and the table settings replaced, the master of ceremonies stepped to the podium and introduced Charles Revson with no reference to what had just occurred. When the waiters brought the food, the curious guests asked what the change was all about. "The

Revlon founder Charles Revson (1906-1975). "[He] had terrible taste in furniture and decor (gold on gold)," said Revlon advertising executive Kay Daly, "but the way a woman should look was native to him."

colors clashed with the room's decor," they were told. Charles Revson had developed a reputation for being able to see subtle variations in shades and hues that others could not, and since his business was based on color, he refused to speak at an event where the colors in the venue clashed. He told the hotel to change the tablecloths or he would not speak.

EARLY SALES EXPERIENCE

Charles Haskell Revson was born on October 11, 1906, outside Boston in the town of Somerville, Massachusetts. He and his two brothers, Joseph and Martin, were raised in nearby Manchester, New Hampshire. Their parents, Samuel and Jeanette, were Russian-born Jews. Jeanette was a saleswoman at a dry-goods store called Nightingales, and Samuel worked for the R. G. Sullivan Company rolling cigars by hand.

Charles was a good student and worked on his school's magazine and yearbook. A talented debater, he helped organize a school debate team. After graduating from Manchester Central High School in 1923, Revson moved to New York and began selling dresses for Pickwick Dress Company. By the time he left the company, he had earned a position as a buyer. This job was more suited to Revson's taste than sales because he enjoyed working with the materials and colors. In 1930, when he was 24, Revson married a young woman named Ida Tompkins, and they moved to Chicago, where he found a job selling sales motivation materials. He did not do well, and the couple, already having marital trouble, moved back to New York. The move did not help the relationship, and they separated and then divorced. At that time Charles's parents had also moved to New York, so he returned home to live with them.

Charles Revson, a Nail Enamel Salesman?

Revson knew he was a good salesman, but his two previous opportunities in sales had not gone well. In 1931, he stumbled into the unlikely position of selling nail enamel for a New Jersey company called Elka. Revson became excited about the possibilities he saw in the nail enamel business. The two people who ran Elka were not very creative businesspeople, but Revson did his homework and found that Elka's product was good. Other enamels or polishes on the market were made with dyes and were transparent, but Elka used a special pigment that really covered the nail.

As he made the rounds selling his product, Revson had an idea that he thought could revolutionize the nail enamel business and make him wealthy. Polishes on the market were available in three shades of red: light, medium, or dark. Revson believed that if Elka's thicker polish was offered in a wider variety of shades, he could capture a huge part of the market. Revson knew he had a winning concept, and he confidently asked his bosses to make his distributorship nationwide so he could take advantage of his idea. To Revson's disappointment, Elka's owners refused to expand his territory. His surprise and frustration did not last long, however, and he realized it was a chance to start his own business.

REVLON OPENS FOR BUSINESS

Revson wasted no time. He and his brother Joseph formed a company with a man named Charles Lachman, whose in-laws owned Dresden, a chemical company that made nail polish and sold it wholesale to other firms. They came up with the name Revlon by inserting the "L" from Lachman's name into their last name. On March 1, 1932, Revlon was officially opened.

Charles Lachman was not particularly adept in the business of color and fashion, so the Revson brothers did almost everything themselves. The nail polish arrived from Dresden in eight-ounce bottles and they would pour it into quarter-ounce bottles, being careful not to spill. This was a tricky job because they had to keep the polish well shaken so all the quarter-ounce bottles would be consistent. To get started, they placed an advertisement in a beauty shop magazine, offering beauticians a bottle of nail polish for 60 cents. They hired someone to pack up the orders and take them to the post office or hand deliver them around town.

As Revlon grew, Revson was able to hire more people and buy equipment. He bought an old filling machine and, according to George Hastell, one of the early employees, it made the filling job much easier. "We put the bottles on wooden trays under a hopper full of four or five gallons of nail enamel," said Hastell. "You pushed a pedal and the filling

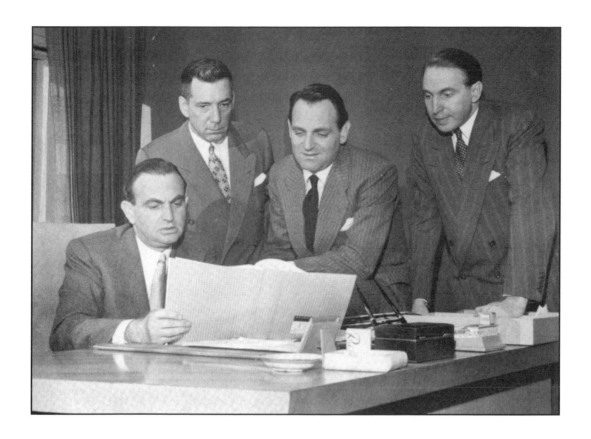

spouts would open up; when the bottles were filled, you'd lift up on the pedal and go to the next row." In 1938, six years after Revlon had opened for business, the company had grown enough that it needed new facilities, and the Revsons moved the small factory to 52nd Street.

The original Revlon partners (left to right): Charles Revson, Charlie Lachman, Martin Revson (who joined in the company in 1935), and Joseph Revson

MOVING OUT OF OBSCURITY

Charles Revson was a perfectionist. Even at this early stage of business when the company counted its pennies, he sometimes threw out batches of nail enamel that were not perfect. He increased the

"All I demand is perfection."
—Charles Revson

variety of colors available, and then monitored their development carefully. Instead of using a color chart as others in the nail polish business did, he actually wore the nail polish on his fingers. He wore the colors all day and observed them under different conditions. His obsession with perfection extended to every area of the business, even applicators. If an applicator brush had any messy bristles, the brush was thrown out. As the company grew larger, Revson implemented quality control checks to ensure the integrity of his products. It would be hard to imagine a business, large or small, that did not have quality control checks today, but in the 1930s Revlon was one of the first.

The first years of operation for Revlon were difficult. Besides being unknown, the company launched its business during the height of the Great Depression. But Revson stuck with his plan to sell nail enamel, working exclusively with beauty salons. He knew that when the manicurists used his polish, they would see the difference in quality and become loyal customers. He was right. News of Revlon nail polish spread by word of mouth and the orders grew larger and larger.

In 1933, Revson had big dreams and a growing company. He could now afford to attend beauty shows as a spectator, although he still could not pay to be an exhibitor at them. While calling on beauty salons, he had met Robert Hoffman, the inventor of the Hoffman professional hair dryer system. Hoffman was a regular exhibitor at beauty shows and offered Revson a corner of his booth. Revson jumped at the chance to demonstrate his products to the attendees, who included retailers, wholesalers, and members of the public. Later, when Revlon became a huge success, Hoffman went to work for the company.

Sales after the first nine months of business were only about $4,000, but the company kept growing. By 1937, Revlon's sales were 40 times greater. Joseph had always taken care of the bookkeeping and managed the plant, and in 1935 Charles's younger brother, Martin, joined the company. Martin took over the sales end of the business, developing a training strategy that would later become standard for teaching salespeople in any industry.

Martin's training method involved having a salesperson act out selling situations in front of a group and then having the group critique him. It sounds simple, but at that time the practice was revolutionary. Although Martin was a tough boss, his sales force grew. The salespeople were aggressive because they knew he did not tolerate lazy workers. One salesman, who was doing poorly, was required to call his sales manager every two hours and report his progress until his performance improved. Revlon's sales team crossed the country, selling to department stores and drugstores as well as beauty salons. Success followed hard work, and the company grew steadily.

REVLON RECEIVES AN "E"

After the devastating economic effects of the Great Depression, America had a new challenge: World

War II. The conflict in Europe began in 1939, and when the United States sent troops to join the effort in 1941, both Martin and Joseph were among them.

Charles received several contracts from the government; therefore, he could support the war effort from home. He created a company called Vorset Corporation in New Jersey to handle the war contracts. His experience with making manicure sets for sale during Christmas promotions and his knowledge of color easily translated into products that could be used by the troops. Vorset made first-aid kits, dye markers that were dropped into the ocean, and even hand grenades. The company did so well in executing the contracts and supporting the U.S. armed forces that in 1944 Revson won the prestigious Army/Navy "E" award, an honor that recognized excellence in production. Later, Revson was able to use his military ties to break into the overseas market by putting his products into military post exchanges.

In addition to his wartime duties, Revson also continued his primary business and added lipsticks to Revlon's product line in 1940. The company had to adapt to stringent conditions when glass bottles were rationed. These bottles and the metal cases used for lipstick were replaced first with plastic and then with paper.

"COPY EVERYTHING"

Charles Revson had a no-fail strategy. With some exceptions, he generally chose not to be the innovator in his field. "Copy everything," he said, "and you can't go wrong." He believed in letting the

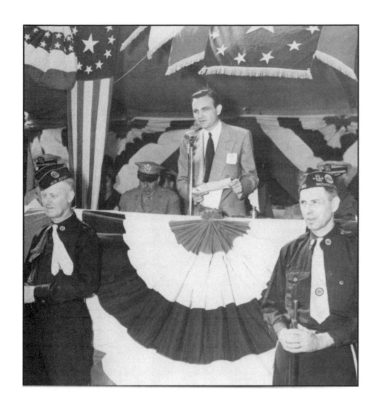

Revson accepting the Army/Navy "E" award in July 1944

competition do the groundwork. When a new product or system was developed, there were always problems to be ironed out. Rather than waste time working to find solutions to these problems, he simply let his competitors do the work. When they came up with a winner, Revson would improve it, put it in a nicer package, and create better advertising.

This approach worked for Revson, but it infuriated his competitors. Estée Lauder reportedly had a saying in her office, "50 percent of Revlon's R and D [Research and Development] is done here." Revson made no apologies for his methods. "I don't think if the competition have got something wonderful, whomever they may be, that there is anything wrong in looking at it, and copying it," he said.

Estée Lauder wasn't the only competitor Revson had his eye on. Madame Helena Rubinstein, whose offices were across the street, would frequently point to the Revlon headquarters and shout, "The Nail Man's busy in there, copying us . . . I swear!"

Revson copied almost everything Estée Lauder did. When she ran black-and-white ads, so did he; when her ads were sepia toned, his were, too. He followed her lead in offering gifts with a purchase, using a single model exclusively, offering a men's fragrance, and naming a fragrance after himself—she created Estée, so he offered Charlie. Just to irritate her, he even put some of the items he copied into his lower-priced lines so they would cheapen her originals. No matter how much he copied Lauder, however, he never captured the high-end market that she did.

Another company Revson borrowed sales techniques from was General Motors, a company he greatly admired. The car manufacturer brought out new colors every fall, and Revson had a semiannual color change with his nail polishes and lipsticks. Since he saw his products as fashion accessories, he encouraged women to wear new shades of polish to match their outfits the way Elizabeth Arden did with her cosmetics. By offering new shades twice per year, he knew women would feel out of style if they did not update their nail polish colors.

Revson also used General Motors as a guide when making his own marketing and organizational decisions. He developed separate cosmetic lines just as GM had separate car divisions. Each cosmetic line focused on a different segment of the market. Revlon was his popularly priced line, Natural Wonder targeted younger women, Moon Drops was for women with dry skin, and Etherea, the hypoallergenic line, helped those with sensitive skin. Etherea was launched in response to Lauder's

Clinique line, introduced in 1968. Revson also offered higher-priced items, such as Marcella Borghese and, at the very top of the line, Ultima II. He used the same marketing techniques with his fragrances, as well.

A MARKETING GENIUS

Revson had a knack for marketing and always tried to find ways to make his products seem more desirable. One way he did this was by carefully balancing supply and demand. During its first five years in business, Revlon sold only to the beauty trade. The customers of department store beauty salons loved Revlon's colors and lasting power so much they began demanding to purchase the products at cosmetics counters. Soon department stores and selected drugstores carried Revlon. This made Revlon's products more widely available, but it also gave them an air of exclusivity.

Revson also invested a large portion of the company's budget in advertising. In the early years, many people thought Revlon was much larger than it actually was because of the volume of advertising. Instead of simply using his ads to describe his products, Revson created a fantasy for his customers. He did not sell red nail polish—he sold "Cherries in the Snow." Revlon's first advertisement in a magazine other than a trade journal was in 1935 in *The New Yorker*. That ad cost the company several hundred dollars—its entire consumer-advertising budget for the year—but by 1975 Revlon was spending $75,000 annually in *The New Yorker*.

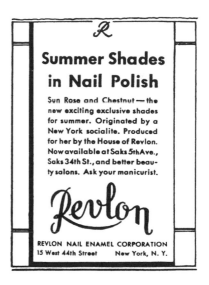

Revlon's first ad in The New Yorker *magazine. It was one-ninth of a page and cost $335.56.*

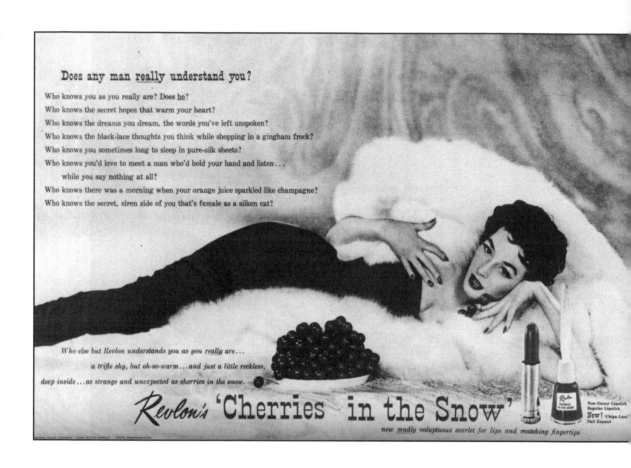

Does any man really understand you?

Who knows you as you really are? Does he?

Who knows the secret hopes that warm your heart?

Who knows the dreams you dream, the words you've left unspoken?

Who knows the black-lace thoughts you think while shopping in a gingham frock?

Who knows you sometimes long to sleep in pure-silk sheets?

Who knows you'd love to meet a man who'd hold your hand and listen . . .
   while you say nothing at all?

Who knows there was a morning when your orange juice sparkled like champagne?

Who knows the secret, siren side of you that's female as a silken cat?

Who else but Revlon understands you as you really are...
   a trifle shy, but oh-so-warm...and just a little reckless,
deep inside...as strange and unexpected as cherries in the snow.

Revlon's 'Cherries in the Snow'

Non-Smear Lipstick
Regular Lipstick
New! 'Chip-Less'
Nail Enamel

new *madly* *voluptuous scarlet for lips and matching fingertips*

"Official spokespeople" are common now, but featuring one model exclusively was quite new when Charles Revson started doing it. In his lifetime, four women—Dorian Leigh, Suzy Parker, Barbara Britton, and Lauren Hutton—were so closely identified with the company that each became known as "the Revlon girl."
This ad features Dorian Leigh.

When Revlon introduced lipsticks that matched the nail polish, the company came out with an ad campaign touting "Matching Lips and Fingertips." The campaign played well in the glossy magazines such as *Vogue*, where ads were in full color and covered two pages. These two-page spreads showed the products attractively, and the message was effective—if women wanted their lips to match their nails, they had to buy both products from Revlon. Revson was not the first in the industry to make use of the matching campaign, but he made it work beautifully.

Another clever marketing strategy Revson used was changing the ratio of product price to the amount of advertising for that product. Originally, Revson would price his items high and then advertise heavily. Under the new strategy, instead of continuing to spend a large amount of money to keep this share of the market, he lowered his advertising for certain products and kept the prices high. Even though sales eventually fell, for a while he earned a large profit.

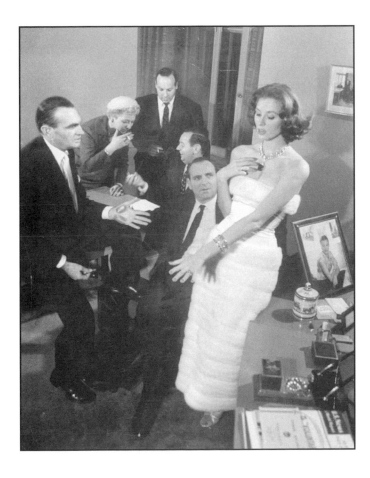

Another Revlon girl, Suzy Parker, was the younger sister of Dorian Leigh. "They don't make combos like that anymore," Revson said of the siblings. Here, Parker examines nail-color samples while Revson tests lipstick shades on the palm of his hand.

The $64,000 Question

When the producers of a new game show, *The $64,000 Question*, were looking for a sponsor in 1955, they were rejected by several major companies. Eventually, producers asked Revlon if it would be interested in sponsoring the TV show. Charles Revson was not fond of television, but one of his competitors, Hazel Bishop, sponsored a different game show and had a competitive edge over Revlon. In order to compete, Revson agreed to sponsor the show.

The first episode of *The $64,000 Question* aired on June 7, 1955, and the program immediately became enormously popular. Movie theaters and restaurants complained the show hurt their business on Tuesday nights because too many people stayed home to watch it. Revlon ads running during the program were so successful that featured items usually sold out within days. Building on the *The $64,000 Question*'s popularity, the producers developed another show as a spinoff—*The $64,000 Challenge*.

Sponsorship of the shows put Revlon well ahead of its close competitors, including Helena Rubinstein and Hazel Bishop. During the live broadcast of *The $64,000 Question*, Revlon had three commercials that were supposed to last one minute each, but they often "accidentally" ran longer. The commercials, like the show, were broadcast live, not taped, so there was no way to shorten them if they ran over the allotted time. This trick gave the company coveted extra commercial time.

The success of *The $64,000 Question* and *Challenge* came to an abrupt halt when a scandal emerged. In a quest for higher ratings, quiz show directors (one of whom, in this case, happened to be Martin Revson, Charles's brother) often fed the answers to the questions to contestants who they, or the sponsors, thought the audience would like to see win. The discovery of this practice led to inquiries about other quiz shows, and these unethical actions were found to have been widespread. It became a huge scandal in the game-show world and many top-dollar shows, whether they were guilty or not, were cancelled. No charges were ever formally brought against the producers of *The $64,000 Question*, but it, like many other game shows, was pulled off the air in 1958.

Not Easy to Live or Work with

Revson worked long hours and expected his staff to do the same. He had a reputation for firing secretaries and top management simply because he did not like something about them. Despite these practices, he was able to attract many talented people over the years because he offered lucrative beginning salaries and benefits. Unfortunately, once they began working for Revlon, employees soon found there was not much room for advancement or for pay increases since they started at such high salaries.

Revson's working relationship with his brothers was not much better than with his top-level employees. Both brothers eventually left Revlon, and they had little contact with Charles afterwards. Charles and Joseph argued about taking the company public. While Charles wanted to do it, Joseph thought it was a bad idea, and in 1955 he left the company. Revlon went public shortly thereafter and was so successful it was listed on the New York Stock Exchange one year later. Martin left in 1958 because he and Charles also had conflicting views about the company's future that they could not resolve.

Revson's personal life was in turmoil, too. He married a total of three times; all the marriages ended in divorce. He had two sons, John and Charles Jr., with his second wife, Johanna Catharina Christina, called Ancky Christina for short. The boys had all the financial benefits of being Charles Revson's sons, but they did not have his time. Even fatherhood could not keep him from putting in many hours at the office.

In the late 1940s, the yearly turnover rate of office staff at Revlon was 166 percent.

going public: offering shares of stock of a privately owned company to the public for the first time

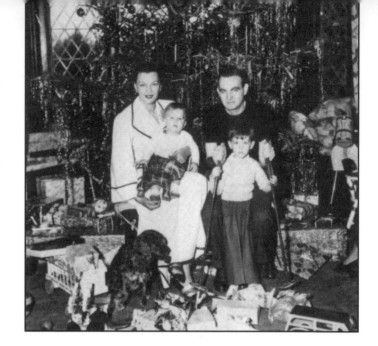

Christmas with Ancky and the boys. Despite the fact that Charles was Jewish, he always gave his children a huge tree and many presents. Sometimes, however, presents aren't enough. Said Charles's son, Charles Revson Jr., "I never really knew my father. I would see him one out of every five or six nights maybe. . . . If anything was wrong, I could always count on his help; but when I was growing up, I didn't see him that much."

His marriage to Ancky did not last, and he married one last time in 1964, to Lyn Sheresky. They divorced in 1974.

LEGACY

Charles Revson died on August 24, 1975, from pancreatic cancer, and Michel Bergerac, head of ITT/Europe, became president of Revlon. In 1985, financier Ron Perelman, one of the the richest people in America, bought the company. In 1999, after some years that saw Revlon losing its market share, Perelman hired Jeffrey Nugent, formerly of Neutrogena, to help turn the company around. The year 2002 saw another change in management as Jack Stahl, who spent more than 20 years at Coca-Cola, took over from Nugent as Revlon's president and chief executive officer.

In spite of losses, Revlon remained, as Stahl said, "One of the most powerful brand names in the world." Known for its nail polish, the company also offered makeup, perfume, and toiletries, and in the 1990s it introduced an innovative product, a transfer resistant lipcolor. This led to a new group of cosmetics all dubbed "transfer resistant," which was called the ColorStay collection. The cosmetics were designed, as the name implies, not to smudge.

The Charles H. Revson Foundation, which Revson established in 1956, was committed to funding ventures connected with urban affairs, education, biomedical research policies, and Jewish philanthropy. During Revson's lifetime he donated $10 million through the foundation, and when he died, he left half his estate to it. Both sons, John and Charles Jr., were active in various roles on the foundation's board of directors. In the twenty-first century, the foundation continued to donate an average of $9 million annually to such projects as *Between the Lions*, a public-television series designed to teach young children to read.

Revlon may have started out to capture the nail enamel market, but the company went on to acquire such recognizable brands and products as Flex hair care, Almay and Ultima II cosmetics, and Charlie, which was the number one fragrance in the world in the 1970s. By 2003, Revlon products could be purchased in 175 countries and territories. Its net sales for 2002 were more than $1.1 billion. Charles Revson's commitment to perfection and eye for color combined to earn his nail enamel company a place as one of America's best-loved brands of mass-market color cosmetics.

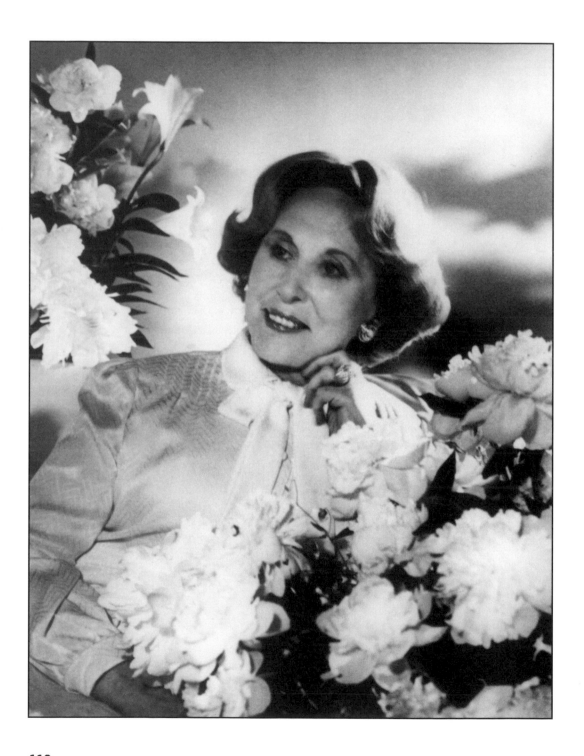

6

ESTÉE LAUDER

DOING BUSINESS
THE ESTÉE WAY

As her friend poured another cup of tea, Estée Lauder excused herself, picked up her purse, and headed for the bathroom. Once inside, she opened her purse and placed several jars on the counter. She picked one up and held it against the wallpaper, then beside the gold-toned faucet, and finally against the peach towels neatly hanging from the hand towel rack. She shook her head, put the jar back into her purse, picked up another, and repeated the ritual. It wasn't until she compared the fourth jar that she smiled, put everything back into her purse, and rejoined her friend.

This unusual exercise was actually Lauder's way of conducting research. She needed new packaging for her increasingly popular cosmetics line, and her first

Energetic and outgoing, Estée Lauder (b. 1908) used her friendly nature and strong family ties to turn her homegrown skin-care business into one of the most recognizable names in the beauty industry.

113

priority was to choose a color and style that would look good in women's bathrooms. Each time she visited a friend, she carried her sample jars with her and compared them to her friend's bathroom. Lauder's company was still small, but her dreams were big and it would not be long before jars in the pleasing blue-green color she selected graced the bathrooms of women all over America.

UNCLE JOHN'S CREAMS

Josephine Esther Mentzer was born in Corona, Queens, New York, on July 1, 1908, although some records say the year of her birth was 1910. Her parents, Rose Schotz Rosenthal Mentzer and Max Mentzer, were both Hungarian Jews who had settled in Corona, where Max opened a hardware store. Rose had been married before and had six children from the first marriage. Josephine—or Esty as her family called her—was Rose's ninth and last child. As a young girl, Esty helped in her father's store and especially loved creating beautiful displays for his windows. She would wrap boxes of nails or tie attractive bows on hammers to show off the store's gift-wrapping. It did not take her long to realize that her father's customers bought more when the items were elegantly displayed. It would be a lesson she would always remember.

As Esty, now calling herself Estée, grew older and started thinking about her future, she showed interest in her uncle's work instead of her father's business. Estée's uncle, John Schotz, was a chemist. He made and sold a number of products such as cold

Estée Lauder was known by various names as a child. Her family seems to have called her Esty, but thanks to her father's accent, school officials misunderstood the spelling of her name, and Esty became "Estée."

creams, fragrances, and lip rouge. (His company, New Way Laboratories, also manufactured such compounds as poultry lice killer, suppositories, and embalming fluid.) She was fascinated watching Uncle John make his cosmetic products, and he taught her to clean her face with his cream instead of harsh soaps and how to do facial massages. She called his cream "Super-Rich All Purpose Creme," and not only did she use it on herself but she also gave it away to all her friends. Estée had a flawless complexion—a perfect advertisement for her uncle's cream—so it was not long before she started selling the cream and some of his other products for him.

THE HOUSE OF ASH BLONDES

After high school, Estée had more time to spend selling her uncle's products, and she focused her interest on the skin-care items he created. By now he had added a few more items to his list of products, which Estée improved and continued to sell to her friends. She also added other items such as eye colors and lipsticks to her inventory.

In her early twenties, Estée fell in love with Joseph Lauter, whom she married on January 15, 1930. They later changed their name to Lauder, which was the original spelling of the family name in Austria, the country from which his parents had emigrated. The couple had a son, Leonard Allan, who was born on March 19, 1933.

As a new mother, Lauder occasionally would treat herself to a visit to the beauty parlor. One day while she was having her hair done at the House of Ash

Blondes, the owner, Florence Morris, asked about her beautiful skin. Lauder was soon back in the salon with samples of the four creams she had been selling. Before Morris knew what she was doing, Lauder was giving her a demonstration of how the products worked. She massaged Morris's skin just the way her uncle taught her, explaining what she was doing with each item. With a flourish she added a final touch of powder and asked Morris what she thought. The demonstration earned Lauder her first job in the beauty business. Morris was opening a new salon and offered Lauder the salon's beauty concession. She would have a small counter in the store where she could sell her products. She would pay

A young Estée Lauder poses for the camera shortly after having her hair done at the House of Ash Blondes.

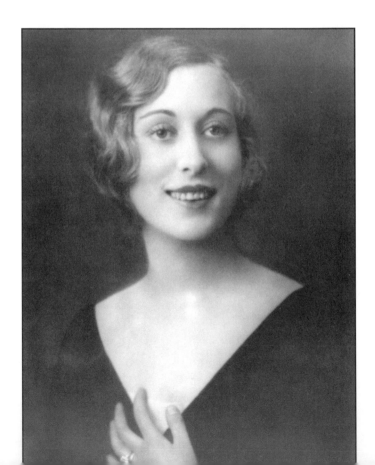

Morris a monthly rent, but the profits from what she sold were hers to keep. Lauder knew it was a huge risk, but she jumped at the opportunity.

When the salon opened for business, so did Estée Lauder's first cosmetics counter. Her display was neatly arranged with black-and-white jars she had bought and hand-lettered with her name. She threw herself into selling her small skin-care line.

THE ESTÉE WAY

Lauder knew from playing in her father's shop as a child that if she wanted someone to buy something, she would have to "sell" it. Morris and her stylists brought the women into the salon, and Lauder took advantage of this captive audience. She waited until the women were placed under the dryer. When they began to get bored, she asked if they would let her try a cream on their faces. When their hair was dry, she would quickly remove the cream and add a touch of rouge (which she called "glow") to their cheeks, some turquoise eye shadow to make the whites of their eyes look whiter, and finally some crimson lipstick. Almost without exception the women were amazed at the effect, enhanced with a new hairstyle. Using this technique, Lauder sold her products to a large number of Morris's customers. She also gave them tiny samples of whatever they did not buy.

Word of mouth spread the news about the cosmetics at Morris's, and before long Lauder had another invitation to demonstrate her products, this time at the Albert and Carter Beauty Salon. She hired and trained a new salesgirl and carefully taught her "the Estée way" of selling. This meant putting the products on the women's skin instead of just talking about them, finishing the look so the women left the salon ready for their next appointments, and always giving a sample of a product they had not purchased. Her clientele grew quickly, and soon women began asking for her products at department stores.

With two concessions and an employee to help, Lauder looked for ways to build up her business. She even made use of her vacation time to promote her products, staying at nice hotels and approaching other female guests to offer facials. She visited women in their homes to show them how to use her products and how to apply color to their faces. She was always perfectly groomed because she knew she had to look successful before other women would be willing to take her advice.

Unfortunately, the energy and drive Estée Lauder poured into building her business meant she was spending less time with her husband, Joe. The troubled relationship fell apart and they divorced in 1939.

GETTING READY FOR THE NEXT LEVEL

Saddened by her divorce, Estée Lauder was more determined than ever to make her business a success. Taking her uncle's advice, she traveled to Miami, the playground of the wealthy, to sell her cosmetics. She set up a concession in a fancy Miami hotel and began traveling back and forth between New York and Miami. In addition to that grueling schedule, she continued to travel to various resorts, building a strong base of customers who loved her products.

Estée enjoyed her work, but she missed Joe. Success meant nothing without him. They rekindled their relationship and were remarried in 1943. Joe left his own business and joined Estée's, where "we would be equal partners in every sense of the word," said Estée. Joe handled financial matters, while Estée concentrated on selling. They welcomed their second son, Ronald, in February 1944. With their family back together, Estée and Joe focused on what needed to be done to move Estée Lauder Cosmetics to the next level of success.

The first thing that had to be revamped was their packaging. The black-and-white bottles and jars did not present the image the Lauders wanted, and the

Estée was known for arriving at parties in Miami bearing a beautifully packaged gift basket of Lauder cosmetics for the hostess.

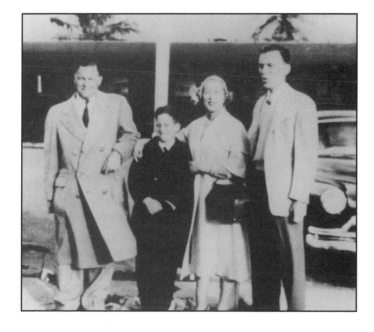

The Lauder family spends some time together in Florida around the late 1950s. Joe, Estée, and Leonard frequently went there on business—and young Ronald got to enjoy the vacations.

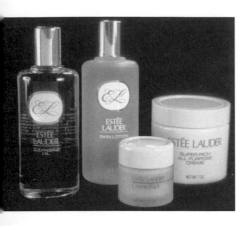

Lauder's first four products, Creme Pack, Cleansing Oil, All Purpose Skin Creme, and Skin Lotion, were immediately well received. Years ahead of their time, the creams and lotions were made with formulas that were still useable more than four decades later. Some of the early products even contained sunscreen for added skin protection.

labels came off in steamy bathrooms. After Estée conducted her informal research to determine a color, they ordered new packaging and bottles for the products.

Next, the Lauders turned their attention to their retail outlets. They knew their products could not compete with other popular cosmetics brands if women could not find them. They needed to get their products into department stores, where larger numbers of women shopped for cosmetics and used their store credit cards—a payment method that often led to more liberal spending. At beauty salons, women typically paid their bills with cash and were less inclined to make spontaneous purchases.

LANDING SAKS FIFTH AVENUE

Estée Lauder had one advantage on her side when approaching the department stores—her customers were already asking where they could purchase her products. In spite of this, it was not easy convincing a large department store to take a risk on her relatively unknown creams and lotions. She was pleased when Bonwit Teller finally agreed to give her some counter space, and she spent every Saturday there selling her cosmetics. But Lauder's ultimate goal was to place her products in Saks Fifth Avenue. The Saks cosmetics buyer, however, saw no need to carry Estée Lauder cosmetics. His customers seemed satisfied with the present cosmetics lines. Besides, Bonwit Teller was already carrying Estée Lauder products, and Saks had a policy of exclusivity.

This was a challenge for Lauder. She needed to prove Saks's customers wanted her products, and she knew exactly how to do it. She was already scheduled to speak to a group of women at a charity luncheon and, as was her custom, she gave out samples of her products. Instead of a small package of cream or a touch of rouge, this time she handed out lipsticks in metal cases, which were almost impossible to get during World War II because of rationing. As she expected, the gifts left an impression on the women and they began requesting her lipsticks at their favorite store—Saks.

This alone may not have been enough to prompt an order from Saks Fifth Avenue, but as luck would have it, Lauder had previously given her Creme Pack treatments to two women associated with Saks. The first woman, Marion Coombs, was an assistant buyer who had scars from a car accident. The second, a daughter of a Saks Fifth Avenue executive, had red blotches on her skin. Both women saw wonderful results from Estée Lauder's creams. When, in 1948, Saks placed its first order of $800, Estée and Joe knew they were on their way to more success. The Saks director of advertising sent out small printed cards with gold lettering that read, "Saks Fifth Avenue is proud to present the Estée Lauder line of cosmetics: now available at our cosmetics department." These cards went to all Lauder's own customers as well as all Saks customers who had charge accounts. The prestige that came with being associated with this department store helped the Lauders launch the products nationally.

For department-store counter openings, Estée developed certain guidelines that she never strayed from: 1) Establish each store herself: train the salespeople, set out the merchandise, create the aura; 2) Choose the right salespeople: intelligent, eager, smiling, and confident; 3) Create attractive counters: mini spas with the elegant blue-green colors; 4) Always offer a gift with purchase.

CONQUERING THE NATION

To fill the Saks order, Estée and Joe opened their first "factory" in a former restaurant and cooked the creams themselves on the stove. They sterilized the jars and bottles, then filled and packaged them for delivery. They worked day and night and only relaxed when the order was delivered in full, and on time. During the next few years, as the company grew, Joe and their older son, Leonard, bottled the products and handled things in the offices, while Estée traveled across the country selling and training

Lauder proudly shows off her first big counter display.

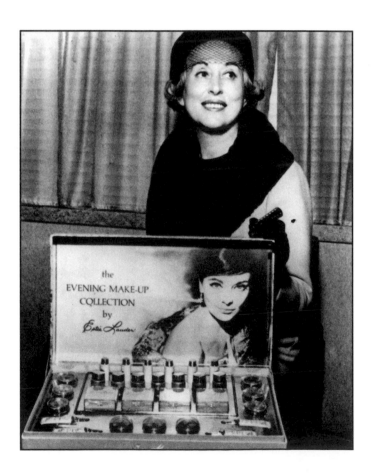

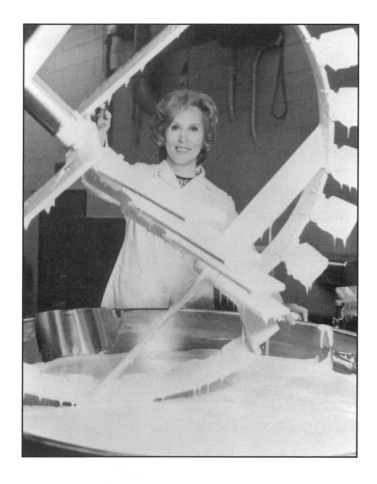

Always involved in every aspect of her company, Lauder is shown here making her products in the company's New York factory.

saleswomen. Account by account, she added to the number of exclusive stores around the country that carried the line, and every extra penny she earned went back into the business.

Everywhere she went, Lauder's energy and natural friendliness helped her build relationships with key people who were in positions to help her. But even so, she had to work hard to finally get Neiman Marcus in Dallas to carry her line in the first years of the 1950s. The store's merchandise manager, Ben Eisner, initially turned her down, but she kept calling him. After several calls he agreed to let her have a small counter with a scheduled opening on New Year's Day, traditionally the worst day to plan an opening. People would have spent all their money buying Christmas presents, and many would still be tired after bringing in the New Year at late-night parties. In addition, it was unusually hot in Dallas, and the store's manager believed no one would show up. Eisner underestimated Lauder, who saw the situation as a wonderful opportunity.

She bought advertising time on a local radio station at 8:15 A.M., January 1 (the station thought no one would be up listening at that hour). Using her most chipper voice she announced, "Good morning, ladies. I'm Estée Lauder just in from Europe with the newest ideas for beauty. In this weather you have to work hard to look your loveliest, and I have the secrets." She described her products and offered a gift for every woman who came to her counter that morning. Then she ended with, "Start the New Year with a new face." The counter was swamped that day, and Lauder was there to stay. For years Neiman Marcus used Lauder's line in their advertisements: "Start the New Year with a New Face . . . Estée Lauder Cosmetics."

Estée Lauder didn't just open counters in stores and then delegate their management; she always thought of new ways to present her products. During a continual whirl of visiting, she would stop in other store departments, such as the hat department, and offer the saleswoman a sample of a lipstick that complemented the color of a special hat. She asked her to mention the Estée Lauder cosmetics

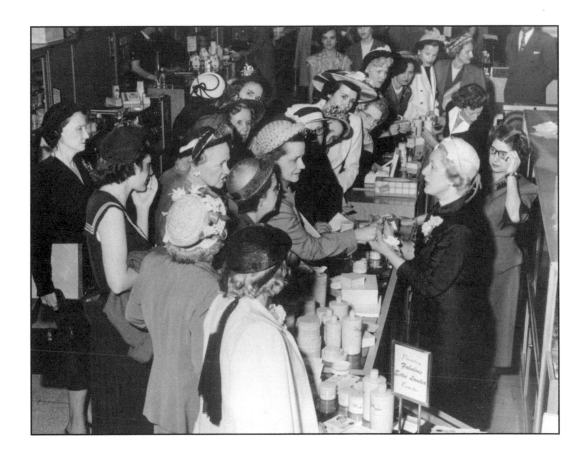

counter to women buying the hats. She also contacted and made friends with all the beauty editors of magazines and newspapers in the towns she visited to make her name known.

YOUTH DEW AND MORE

Lauder's hard work at marketing her cosmetics made her business profitable, but it was the introduction in 1953 of her bath oil, Youth Dew, that catapulted her to phenomenal success. The oil was poured into a woman's bath. The scent clung to her body long

A sign said that this department store was pleased to be "Presenting Fabulous Estée Lauder Cosmetics." In this case, the store also presented Lauder herself. Here, she demonstrates her cosmetics on eager customers.

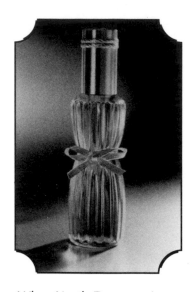

When Youth Dew was introduced at Bonwit Teller in 1953 as a gift with purchase, many women bought Lauder's skin-care line just so they could have the Youth Dew gift. Youth Dew's success was phenomenal—especially because Lauder did almost no advertising for the product aside from enticing customers with the scent by wearing it everywhere.

hyaluronic acid: a gelatinous substance found in the eyes, joint fluid, and the spaces between tissues that acts as a lubricant and protective agent

after she was dressed and moving through her day, in effect doubling as a perfume. Later, Youth Dew was developed into a perfume as well.

With the amazing response to Youth Dew, Estée Lauder products became the cosmetics of choice for many wealthy women. When Re-Nutriv Cream, touted to have anti-aging qualities, was introduced in 1957, the retail price of $115 per pound and the full-page advertisement in *Harper's Bazaar* made it clear which customers Lauder was targeting. When she advertised her products, Lauder used a single model over a period of time so her customers could see how the products worked with one person's skin as she aged. One extremely well-received campaign used the model Karen Graham. Graham's face became so associated with Estée Lauder cosmetics that many people thought she was actually Estée Lauder herself.

LEGACY

After years of working closely with his parents starting in 1958, Leonard Lauder became chief executive officer of the company in 1982, a position he held until 1999. Under his leadership, the company focused on research and development, working with two labs that were researching skin-cell repair and the use of hyaluronic acid as a moisture preserver. Out of this research came one of the company's most successful skin-care formulations, Night Repair. In 1999, Fred H. Langhammer was promoted to president and chief executive officer of The Estée Lauder Companies.

Ronald Lauder, Estée's younger son, joined the family business in 1964 and went on to become chairman of Clinique laboratories, a position he continued to hold in 2003. In 1986, President Ronald Reagan appointed Ronald Lauder U.S. ambassador to Austria. While in Europe, he became more aware of the horrific effects of the Holocaust, during which countless numbers of Jews were exterminated in German concentration camps. His experience led him to create the Ronald S. Lauder Foundation, dedicated to helping revitalize Jewish communities in Eastern and Central Europe that were devastated by the Holocaust.

Ronald was following the example of his parents, who had created the Estée and Joseph Lauder Foundation, Inc., in 1962. The foundation built parks for children in New York City, providing badly needed places for children to play safely. The parks were called "adventure playgrounds" and designed to excite the children's imaginations. The foundation also funded art museums and Jewish causes.

Among the many awards Estée Lauder received was France's Legion of Honor in 1978, for contributing financially to the restoration of the Palace of Versailles. Another honor came when President Richard Nixon offered her the ambassadorship to Luxembourg. Though thrilled with the offer, she declined.

Joseph Lauder died in 1983, on the couple's 53rd anniversary of their first wedding. After working together for so long to build their business, it took Estée some time to recover from Joe's death.

Clinique

In the 1960s, there was a growing criticism that makeup and the way it was marketed were demeaning to women. Estée Lauder responded in 1968 by introducing a new line of modestly priced products called Clinique, aimed at younger woman "to whom beauty was less embellishment than fitness, health, and good caretaking." The company focused the line's advertising on caring for and protecting the skin. Clinique was fragrance-free and allergy-tested, and it was based on a dermatologist's view of the future of skin care: cleanse (with soap and water), clear with a clarifier, and moisturize. It was easy and no-nonsense.

Photographs showed the products rather than the women using them. One long-running advertisement showed a toothbrush in a glass next to Clinique products, with the words "twice a day." Like brushing the teeth, cleansing, clarifying, and moisturizing with Clinique were to be a part of a daily routine. The Clinique store counters presented a contrasting image to other makeup counters in department stores. A combination of antiseptic green packaging and florescent-lighted counter space created an air of no-nonsense sterility aimed at young professionals, as did the Clinique beauty consultants, who wore white lab coats. Many businesswomen and feminists who might not have felt comfortable using traditional beauty products used Clinique cosmetics.

Clinique was actually Leonard Lauder's idea. As he explained, "The reason we launched Clinique is that I felt that if I were going to go into business against Estée Lauder this is exactly how I would do it."

More than 50 years after Estée and Joe first cooked creams on a stove in their small factory, Estée Lauder Cosmetics had become The Estée Lauder Companies, one of the leading manufacturers and marketers of prestige skin-care, makeup, fragrance, and hair-care products in America. The company launched such successful brands as Clinique, Origins (cosmetics based on natural ingredients), and Aramis (colognes and after-shaves for men). Lauder's Re-Nutriv Cream remained hugely successful and generated other anti-aging Re-Nutriv products. In the 1990s, the company began to expand by purchasing such brands as Bobbi Brown Essentials cosmetics and Aveda.

In 2002, The Estée Lauder Companies posted annual sales of almost $5 billion, marking over 50 years of uninterrupted growth. It sold its products in more than 130 countries and territories worldwide, and also licensed many other well-known brands such as Tommy Hilfiger and Donna Karan fragrances. The Estée Lauder Companies went public on the New York Stock Exchange in 1995, but Lauder family members continued to help guide the company, building on Estée Lauder's reputation for offering elegantly marketed, quality products.

Lauder had a "hands-on" approach to business. Here she demonstrates her cosmetics on department-store customers.

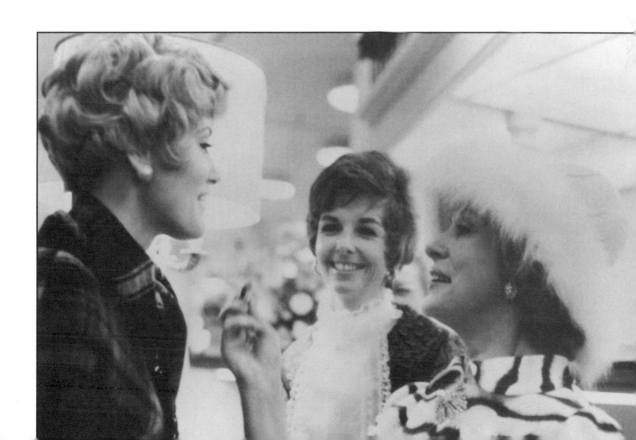

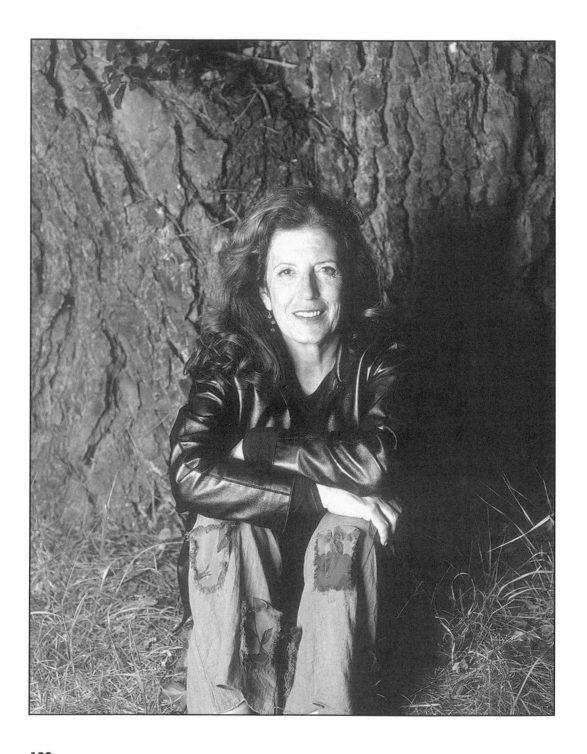

7

ANITA RODDICK

REVOLUTIONIZING THE COSMETICS INDUSTRY

The classroom was filled with children waiting for their lesson to begin. They watched every move of their teacher, Anita Perella, knowing she would have something exciting and totally unexpected planned. Today's subject was medieval history, and they had already read their assigned chapter. But instead of taking out her textbook, Perella took out a record player. Soon low sounds filled the classroom. "This is a Gregorian chant," she began, and as the chant rose and fell, she brought to life the words they had read in their books.

Anita Perella might have gone on to retire as the most popular teacher in her school, but instead she became known for revolutionizing the cosmetics industry. She never lost her penchant for creativity

"For [The Body Shop], beauty is a healthy part of everyday life," said founder Anita Perella Roddick (b. 1942). "It's all about character and curiosity and imagination and humor—in short, it's an active, outward expression of everything you like about yourself."

and made it an important element in her company, The Body Shop.

LITTLEHAMPTON

Anita Perella was born in Littlehampton, on the south coast of England, on October 23, 1942. Her mother, Gilda, was born in Italy and moved to England as a nanny when she was 15. Anita's father, Henry Perella, was Gilda's second husband. Anita, her two older half-sisters, Lydia and Velia, and her brother, Bruno, learned early about hard work, helping out in the Clifton Café owned by their parents. Later, her father converted the café into an American-style ice-cream soda shop, putting in pinball machines and a jukebox and offering exotic ice-cream sundaes and Coca-Cola. The family's café became one of Littlehampton's favorite places for young people to hang out. Anita paid attention. By adding a little drama to completely change the café's atmosphere, her father had created a successful business out of a floundering one. He died of a heart attack when Anita was only 10.

After high school, Anita thought seriously about becoming an actress, but she followed her mother's advice and went to teacher-training college instead. Anita taught school for a while but, even though she loved her job, she knew she wanted to travel. In 1962, she had visited Israel on a scholarship and worked in a kibbutz on the shores of Lake Tiberias. This amazing experience made her long for the world outside the classroom, so she left her teaching position and traveled to Geneva, where she spent a

"Be special, be anything but mediocre."
—Gilda Perella's advice to her daughter Anita

kibbutz: a collective farm in Israel

year working for the United Nations. She then traveled to exotic locations such as Tahiti, Australia, South Africa, Madagascar, and Mauritius before returning to England. She experienced a different adventure when she returned to Littlehampton. Her mother introduced her to Gordon Roddick, and she fell in love. Before long they were married while on a trip to the United States.

ENTERING THE BUSINESS WORLD

With one child, Justine, and another on the way, Gordon and Anita decided they wanted to have a business of their own to run together. They bought an old Victorian house in Littlehampton and ran it as

Anita and Gordon Roddick

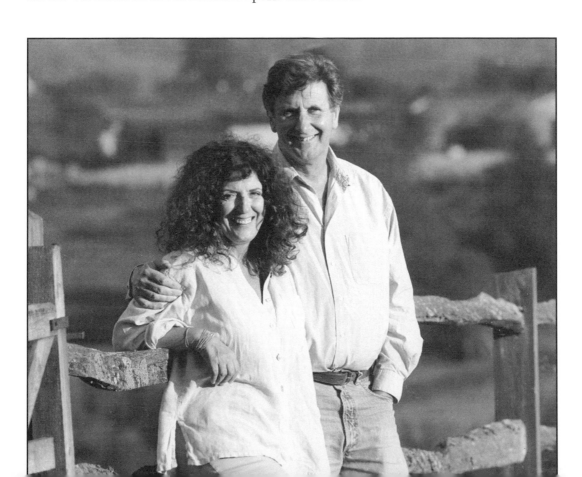

a bed-and-breakfast, but when the summer ended the guests stopped arriving and their income suddenly dried up. Forced to make a decision, they turned half the bed-and-breakfast into a residential hotel, where customers could rent a room year-round. To supplement their income, they opened a restaurant called Paddington's, but their original plan to serve health foods did not go over well. So they turned the restaurant into an American-style burger joint and added loud rock music. The changes energized the business overnight. Paddington's became a hot spot.

The Roddicks ran the restaurant and hotel for three years before deciding it was simply too much work and they needed to make a change. At this time, Gordon told Anita about his dream—to go on a two-year horseback expedition from Buenos Aires to New York! Once she recovered from the surprise, Roddick supported his decision, but she knew she needed something to provide for herself and their two girls, Justine and Samantha, while he was gone. They still had the residential hotel, but she needed something else to pay the bills.

SKIN CARE LEADS TO THE BODY SHOP

The Roddicks brainstormed about the kind of business Anita might enjoy running while still spending time with the girls. She had picked up a lot of information about skin and hair care during her travels, and it did not take her long to decide to sell beauty products. Her products would use natural ingredients, such as the cocoa butter Tahitian women used as a moisturizer. Additionally, she would offer her products in smaller sizes, so women would not have to buy more than they really needed. She read all she could about making cosmetics, from grandmothers' secrets to books on kitchen cosmetics. She experimented with these recipes by trying them on her own skin, but soon realized she needed help. After looking in the telephone book's yellow pages under "herbalist," Roddick found a chemist who was willing to work with her. Together they came up with about 25 products using ingredients like aloe vera, jojoba, and almond oil.

Roddick chose to open her store in Brighton, which was 20 miles away from Littlehampton. Brighton was more upscale, yet it was popular with hippies who would love her natural ingredients. The building she found was in Kensington Gardens—a slightly run-down area, but one that still had a lot of pedestrian shopping. She paid six months' rent in advance and began to prepare the store for the opening.

To create packaging, Roddick bought a supply of the type of inexpensive containers that hospitals used to collect urine samples. As cheap as they were, she still could not afford to buy as many as she thought she would need. Instead, she would tell her customers to bring their containers back for refills. She and her friends hand-labeled the first bottles and filled them with the products in her kitchen. Some of the cosmetics were so new, Roddick wrote the ingredients down on postcards for the customers,

While in America, Roddick had seen "body shops," where car bodies were repaired after accidents. When she was deciding on a name for her store, the name "The Body Shop" seemed a perfect fit.

135

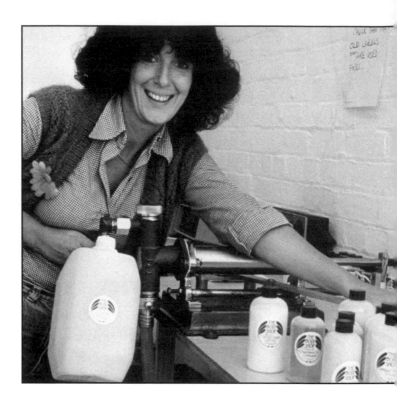

Roddick bottling some of The Body Shop's earliest products

Shortly before the store was to open, Roddick received a letter from two neighboring funeral parlors threatening to sue her. They claimed their business would be affected because people whose loved ones had recently died would not hire a funeral director with offices next to a "Body Shop." Roddick went to the newspapers with her story, and the press coverage she received made good free advertising.

adding information about where the contents came from and what they would do.

DIFFERENT FROM THE REST

The store opened in March 1976, and from the very beginning it was clear: The Body Shop was to be different from previous cosmetic stores. In other stores, the salespeople were trained to persuade the customers to purchase as much as they could. But in The Body Shop, customers were never pressured to buy items they could not afford and were encouraged to bring in their own containers. Instead of a one-year or five-year business plan, all Anita had was a guideline from Gordon. He told her she would need to earn 300 pounds (about $475) in sales per week to make ends meet, and that became her goal. When she did not make her goal, she kept the shop open late, opened on Sundays, or took a selection of products to schools or evening institutes to try to earn more.

Choosing to open her first store in Brighton turned out to be a good idea. The store did well in its first year of business, partly because the hot weather brought more tourists. Women who liked to show off their skin loved the natural lotions and other skin-care products sold by The Body Shop. Roddick knew her idea was popular long before the first year was over, and she decided to open a second shop. This time she chose Chichester, a yachting

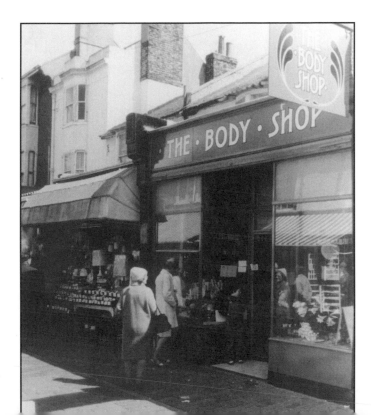

The original The Body Shop in Brighton, England

town about the same distance from Littlehampton as Brighton. The Chichester shop opened for business in September 1976.

Soon after this opening, Roddick met an herbalist named Mark Constantine who made quality products with all-natural ingredients. Unfortunately, the products looked terrible and smelled even worse. He had a lettuce lotion that had bits of lettuce floating in it and a honey and beeswax cleanser with black specks from the bees' dirty feet. Roddick saw potential, however. If she bought his products and wrote out little cards explaining why the products looked the way they did, as well as what they would do for customers' skin, she thought she could sell them.

The Chichester, England, storefront. To get the money to open her second shop, Roddick accepted a loan of about $6,000 from a friend's boyfriend. In exchange, she gave him half the business. For Ian McGlinn, the investor, this loan turned into $6.4 million when The Body Shop went public in 1984. By 2002, his investment was worth about $72 million.

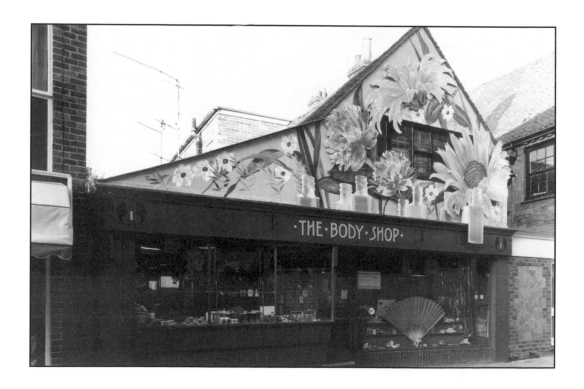

She was right, and by the time Gordon returned home from South America, both shops were doing well. The Roddicks sold the hotel to focus on The Body Shop, and Gordon took over bottling and delivering the products and handling the books. In 1977, they opened their third store and moved Gordon's bottling operation to an old furniture depository in Littlehampton.

The Body Shop was thriving. Determined to learn about the industry they were operating in, Anita Roddick went to conferences and presentations given by other cosmetics companies, such as Estée Lauder and Revlon. She soon realized that she did not want to do business the way they did. "I did not speak the same language as these people, I did not even look like them—all the other women were in silk and furs, while I was in jeans," she said.

Meanwhile, Gordon had been thinking about The Body Shop's future. He realized there was a way to open more shops without having to come up with financing for the ventures. Many of their friends and customers wanted to open their own store, so Gordon came up with something he called "self-financing." The Roddicks believed self-financing was an original idea, but the concept was actually the same as franchising. People could open shops and use the name "The Body Shop." In exchange for using the name, they had to agree to sell the Roddicks' products. In the beginning, Anita and Gordon did not charge franchise fees because they hoped the increase in sales would allow them to buy their ingredients in bulk for less and increase their profit margin. The first informal franchise opened in 1978.

GROWTH LEADS TO ACTIVISM

The Roddicks' bottling operation soon outgrew the furniture depository and in October 1982 they moved into a new warehouse and office complex they had built in Littlehampton using money from a bank loan. New shops were opening at the rate of two each month, with shops in Iceland, Denmark, Finland, and the Netherlands. They began charging a franchise fee and created rules about what could and could not be done in the shops. Rather than using traditional advertising, they hired a public-relations person to come up with creative ways to promote the company. During one London Marathon when runners complained about sore feet, The Body Shop employees handed out free samples of peppermint foot lotion along the route. The foot lotion became a best-selling product.

The Roddicks also drew attention to their company through activism. In 1985, they sponsored posters for Greenpeace's campaign against dumping hazardous waste in the North Sea. It was the first time the environmental group had joined hands with a commercial company. Another campaign, this one against the slaughter of whales, was more direct. Many cosmetics companies used whale oil in their creams. It was almost identical to jojoba oil, made from a desert plant that some Native Americans had been using in their hair and on their skin for years. Anita wanted to convince the cosmetics companies,

The Body Shop did not test on animals. When testing was required, it used human volunteers from the staff or from a clinic in England.

as well as consumers, to use jojoba instead of sperm whale oil, so she sponsored the campaign.

Many of the ingredients the Roddicks used came from economically distressed areas. The Body Shop developed a system of community trade links that allowed poor families around the world to find employment while providing The Body Shop with products it needed. Among the products acquired through trade links were sesame seed oil from a village in Nicaragua, shea nut butter from Ghana, and oil from Brazil nuts found in the Amazon rain forest. The Roddicks also found resources closer to home in Easterhouse, a town near Glasgow, Scotland. When the Roddicks visited the area, there were no places for

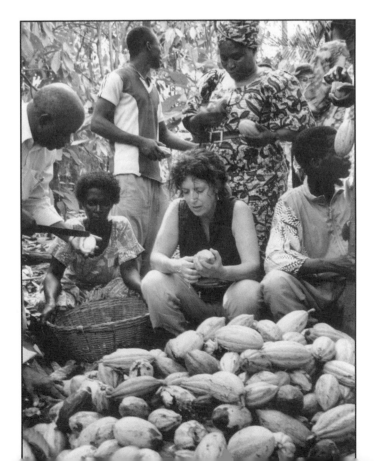

Roddick and cocoa farmers from the Kuapa Kokoo Cooperative in Ghana process cocoa beans. The Body Shop uses these beans to produce its moisturizing cocoa butter.

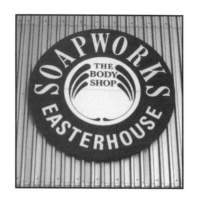

The sign outside The Body Shop Easterhouse Soapworks factory near Glasgow, Scotland

the children to play and no jobs for their parents. Gordon came up with the idea to help the community by building a factory to make soaps for The Body Shop. The Roddicks made a commitment to the townspeople that 25 percent of the profits from the soap sales would be used to help rebuild the community. The factory employed many of the townspeople, and the profits from the soap sales were used for many projects, including the construction of a new playground. Easterhouse became a thriving community.

In April 1984, The Body Shop became a publicly owned company and the Roddicks were instant millionaires. By 2000, there were almost 1,800 shops in 49 markets, doing business in 24 languages. Gordon and Anita knew chasing profits was not their style and wanted to use their status for something meaningful. They decided to continue to use The Body Shop to raise the public consciousness.

CARING FOR EMPLOYEES AND COMMUNITIES

Doing business in a nontraditional way (focusing on helping communities rather than on making a profit) also translated into treating employees differently. Unlike many other companies, The Body Shop discouraged hierarchies among its employees. The Roddicks felt it was important to know what their employees were thinking and what issues within the company they disliked, so they developed the "red letter" system. Employees could write their complaints down, put them in a red envelope, mail them to a board member, and they would receive a response in 24 hours. The red-letter system helped identify weaknesses in the company's maternity benefits program, and the program was adjusted in response to the complaints. On another occasion, employees had a chance to see Anita's commitment to addressing their needs. The Body Shop employees wore uniforms that changed about four times a year. Employees did not like one uniform, which included bright red culottes, and when Anita visited some of the stores, they told her about their dislike. Her response was immediate, "Parcel them up and send them to me." She found a group in Romania that was able to use the culottes. On another occasion, Anita walked into a store and saw several

Roddick saw The Body Shop personnel as members of a team, rather than a hierarchy of employees. She would frequently visit with, and work alongside of, staff members at franchise stores all over the world. Here, she is behind the counter of the Kensington store celebrating the company's 25th anniversary.

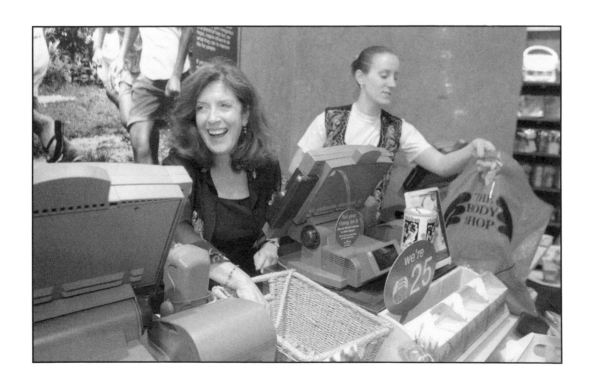

"There aren't many motivating forces more potent than giving your staff an opportunity to exercise and express their idealism."
—Anita Roddick

employees wearing crumpled shirts. When she spoke to them about their appearance, they said, "You're assuming we all have washing machines and ironing boards, like you." They were right, she had assumed that, so she made sure all staff rooms had an iron and ironing board available for employees.

In 1985, The Body Shop Training School opened in London. It was a corporate training school, but it was very different from the usual corporate training schools, which focused on raising profits. Instead, its focus was on human development, consciousness-raising, and product knowledge. For example, the school ran seminars on drug and alcohol abuse and environmental issues. In 1987, The Body Shop created a video production company called Jacaranda Productions to create training videos, weekly television information, and documentary programs.

Toward the end of the 1990s, the Roddicks and their top management staff decided to shift the company's focus from manufacturing and distributing its products to sales and marketing. The cost and time involved in manufacturing and distribution had caused the retail price—the price paid in the store by its customers—to be unnecessarily high. Solving this problem meant reorganizing the company and it also meant letting many employees go. Anita and Gordon were heartbroken, but they knew it had to be done and they decided to downsize as humanely as possible. Employees and even members of their families were offered training in new skills, and those who wanted to open their own businesses received help through the entrepreneur's club. Everyone who left had full use of company facilities, from the childcare center to the gym, for another nine months.

Anita and Gordon knew many of their employees shared their passion for helping others, so they set up the Community Care Department. Through this department, stores could contribute to the community in which they were located. Employees became involved in such projects as the Avon Wildlife Trust, where they helped run an educational training establishment and a demonstration organic farm. Another store sponsored a full-time warden for the Northamptonshire Wildlife Trust.

BUILDING A BUSINESS IN AMERICA

Americans who visited Britain and bought The Body Shop products wondered why there were no stores in the United States. The company received thousands of letters asking for The Body Shop in America. In 1988, The Body Shop finally entered the American market and found business there different from what the Roddicks were used to. Franchising meant the company did not have enough of a profit margin to offer discounts, but Americans were used to sales and "gifts with purchase"—promotions The Body Shop had never used. Also, the company's strong commitment to activism tended to make Americans, who were not used to mixing politics with retailing, uncomfortable. Opening in the U.S. forced the Roddicks to look at ways to adapt to a new market. As a result, the company moved away from franchising because some shops had differing opinions about how to operate a business, and some franchises did

Testing on animals in the cosmetics industry has often included cruel practices such as dropping hair-care products into rabbits' eyes, and force-feeding rats shampoo until they die to determine levels of toxicity. Disgusted with such practices, The Body Shop collected four million signatures in a single year to protest. In November 1998, the United Kingdom introduced a ban on animal testing for cosmetics.

In 1990, The Body Shop hired an anthropologist, becoming the first cosmetics company to do so. The scientist researched, and then catalogued, disappearing tribes' histories, as well as information about their traditional methods of skin care and hair care.

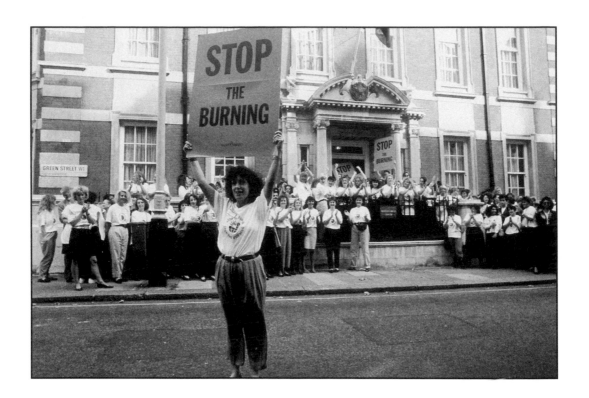

Outside the Brazilian embassy in England, Roddick protests the burning of rain forests.

not always maintain The Body Shop's high standards. In order to regain some control over its image and reduce unnecessary costs, The Body Shop began to buy back some franchises and entered into a partnership arrangement with others.

LEGACY

Once they realized how successful The Body Shop could be, Anita and Gordon Roddick were determined to show the world that a thriving corporation could do business ethically. When they started, their commitment to using their position and profits to create a better world was considered new and different. A number of their competitors copied their products, but none copied their way of doing business and their political activism. Anita Roddick believed that was because The Body Shop did not put profit making first. The company's commitment to activism, however, gave it a recognizable identity and motivated the employees. "I think that is more engaging and more meaningful than any advertising campaign," she said.

Other cosmetics firms tried to convince consumers makeup is essential, but Roddick said, "No one *needs* anything we sell. . . . None of our products are a matter of life and death, so campaigning for me became the method by which we could introduce values into a nonvalue industry."

Over the years, the buying public embraced The Body Shop products. In 2002, the company estimated that its 77 million customers made a purchase from one of The Body Shop stores every 0.4 seconds.

The Body Shop continually looked at ways to remain competitive. It launched The Body Shop at Home, which used the in-home method of direct selling. Roddick saw exploring different avenues of doing business as a way to launch new products and promote activism and environmental issues.

In 2002, Anita Roddick announced she would step down as head of the company in order to focus her attention entirely on activism. She felt she had created a model for others to follow. From one store in 1976 to 1,954 stores and more than $1 billion in annual sales reported in 2002, Anita and Gordon's success far exceeded their dreams. Many people said business could not be conducted the way the Roddicks did it, but The Body Shop became one of Britain's largest international retailers, and proved them wrong.

"The plain truth is, no cosmetic product can prevent the aging process. . . . Any product that could do that would not be a cosmetic, it would be a drug."
—Anita Roddick

GLOSSARY

alpha-hydroxy acid: a group of fruit-based acids that trap moisture in the skin and can help stimulate new tissue growth; often used in wrinkle creams

apothecary: a person who prepares and sells drugs and medicines; a pharmacist

astringent: a substance that causes tissues in the body to constrict or draw together

cold cream: a cream used for cleaning and softening the skin

cosmetic: a product applied to the face, hair, or body that is designed to beautify the wearer, or to cover up a blemish or defect. Face powder, lipstick, and rouge are examples of cosmetics.

damask: a heavy fabric of cotton, silk, linen, or wool woven with elaborate patterns

direct sales: the sale of goods from one individual to another, often done door-to-door or in the customer's home. Avon products and Girl Scout cookies are examples of products sold by direct sales.

eye shadow: a cosmetic applied to the eyelids to enhance the eyes

franchise: a licensing arrangement in which an investor pays money to the owner of a particular brand-name product or business for permission to sell that product or operate that business in a certain territory. The person offering permission is called the **franchiser**. The person buying the rights is the **franchisee**.

going public: offering shares of stock of a privately owned company to the public for the first time

greasepaint: a type of theatrical makeup, usually made by combining a preparation of grease with colors

haute couture: (from French, meaning "high or elegant sewing") fashion created exclusively for one person; also the designers or establishments that create this fashion

hyaluronic acid: a gelatinous substance found in the eyes, joint fluid, and the spaces between tissues that acts as a lubricant and protective agent

hypoallergenic: products designed to have a decreased tendency to cause an allergic reaction

jojoba: a shrub with leathery leaves and edible seeds, which contain an oil commonly used in cosmetics and also as a lubricant

kibbutz: a collective farm in Israel

mascara: a cosmetic applied to the eyelashes to darken them

mass production: the manufacture of goods in large quantities

New York Stock Exchange: the oldest and largest stock exchange in the U.S., established in 1792. Located on Wall Street in New York City, the NYSE trades more than 2,600 stocks, and each company must meet the exchange's strict listing requirements.

patent: the exclusive right to produce and sell a certain product or invention

pheromone: a chemical given off by an animal or person that can influence the behavior of other members of the species, frequently used to attract a mate

retail: selling goods in small amounts directly to customers. Wal-Mart and Target are examples of retail stores.

rouge: a type of cosmetic, usually red or pink in color, applied to the lips or cheeks

shareholder: a person who owns a portion of a company, in the form of shares of stock

stock market: an organized market where stocks and bonds are actively traded

toiletries: articles used in personal grooming, such as toothpaste and hair spray

trade show: an exhibition where people from a particular industry gather together to display and look at the latest products and technology in their field

wholesale: selling goods in bulk, or in large quantities, usually done from the manufacturer to the retail store

witch hazel: a solution made from the bark and leaves of the witch hazel shrub and used as an astringent

BIBLIOGRAPHY

"About Helena Rubinstein." http://www.helenarubinstein.com/_int/_en/aboutHR/abouthr.aspx.

Adams, Russell B., Jr. *King C. Gillette, The Man and His Wonderful Shaving Device*. Boston: Little, Brown, 1978.

"All About Avon." http://www.avoncompany.com/about/.

Angeloglou, Maggie. *A History of Make-up*. New York: Macmillan, 1970.

Basten, Fred E. *Max Factor's Hollywood: Glamour, Movies, Make-up*. Santa Monica, Calif.: W. Quay Hays, 1995.

"Charles H. Revson Foundation." http://www.revsonfoundation.org/about_chr.htm.

"The Company For Women." http://www.avoncompany.com/women/.

"Creative Quotations from Helena Rubinstein." http://creativequotations.com/one/1402.htm.

"Elizabeth Arden: Our Heritage." http://www.elizabetharden.com/heritage/early_start.asp.

Gere, Charlotte, and Marina Vaizey. *Great Women Collectors*. London: Philip Wilson, 1999.

"Gillette at a Glance." http://www.gillette.com/company/gilletteataglance.asp.

Harris, Jessica B. *The World Beauty Book: How We Can All Look and Feel Wonderful Using the Natural Beauty Secrets of Women of Color*. New York: HarperSanFrancisco, 1995.

"Helena Rubinstein Foundation." http://fdncenter.org/grantmaker/rubinstein/.

"Helena Rubinstein Foundation: About Helena Rubinstein." http://fdncenter.org/grantmaker/rubinstein/about.html.

Hinds, Patricia Mignon. *The Essence Total Makeover: Body, Beauty, Spirit*. New York: Crown, 1999.

Israel, Lee. *Estée Lauder: Beyond the Magic*. New York: Macmillan, 1985.

Lauder, Estée. *Estée: A Success Story*. New York: Random House, 1985.

Lewis, Alfred Allan, and Constance Woodworth. *Miss Elizabeth Arden: An Unretouched Portrait*. New York: Coward, McCann & Geoghegan, 1972.

McConnell, D. H., Sr. *Great Oak: A History of the California Perfume Company*. New York: Avon Products, Inc., 1978.

McHenry, Robert. *Famous American Women: A Biographical Dictionary from Colonial Times to the Present.* New York: Dover, 1980.

"Max Factor's Heritage." http://www.maxfactor.com/uk/.

"Maybelline: Early Successes." http://www.maybelline.com/us/success.html.

Moskowitz, Milton, Robert Levering, and Michael Katz. *Everybody's Business: A Field Guide to the 400 Leading Companies in America.* New York: Doubleday, 1990.

O'Higgins, Patrick. *Madame: An Intimate Biography of Helena Rubinstein.* New York: Viking, 1971.

Peiss, Kathy. *Hope in a Jar: The Making of America's Beauty Culture.* New York: Metropolitan, 1998.

Pinckney, Gerrie, and Marge Swenson. *New Image for Women.* New York: Swenson & Pinckney, 1987.

"Revlon Corporate." http://www.revlon.com/corporate/.

Roddick, Anita. *Body and Soul: Profits with Principles, the Amazing Success Story of Anita Roddick and The Body Shop.* New York: Crown, 1991.

———. *Business as Unusual.* London: Thorsons, 2000.

"Stahl Succeeds Nugent as Revlon President, CEO." http://www.chaindrugreview.com/articles/Stahl_succeeds_Nugent.html.

Tobias, Andrew. *Fire and Ice: The Story of Charles Revson—the Man Who Built the Revlon Empire.* New York: William Morrow, 1975.

Wells, Reggie, and Theresa Foy DiGeronimo. *Face Painting: African American Beauty Techniques from an Emmy Award-Winning Makeup Artist.* New York: Henry Holt, 1998.

SOURCE NOTES

Quoted passages are noted by page and order of citation.

Introduction

p. 15: Kathy Peiss, *Hope in a Jar: The Making of America's Beauty Culture* (New York: Metropolitan, 1998), 55.

p. 22: Patricia Mignon Hinds, *The Essence Total Makeover: Body, Beauty, Spirit* (New York: Crown, 1999), 10.

Chapter One

pp. 32-33: D. H. McConnell Sr., *Great Oak: A History of the California Perfume Company* (New York: Avon Products, Inc., 1978), 10.

p. 38: McConnell, *Great Oak*, 13.

Chapter Two

p. 41 (caption): Patrick O'Higgins, *Madame: An Intimate Biography of Helena Rubinstein* (New York: Viking, 1971), 144.

p. 41: "Creative Quotations from Helena Rubinstein, "http://creativequotations.com/one/1402.htm.

p. 42 (margin): O'Higgins, *Madame*, 19.

p. 46 (caption): O'Higgins, *Madame*, 42.

p. 52 (first margin): O'Higgins, *Madame*, 47.

p. 52 (second margin): O'Higgins, *Madame*, 48.

p. 52 (third margin): O'Higgins, *Madame*, 50.

p. 52 (first): Alfred Allan Lewis and Constance Woodworth, *Miss Elizabeth Arden: An Unretouched Portrait* (New York: Coward, McCann & Geoghegan, 1972), 86.

p. 52 (second): O'Higgins, *Madame*, 70.

p. 52 (third): Lewis, *Miss Elizabeth Arden*, 86.

p. 53: "Gillette at a Glance," http://www.gillette.com/company/gilletteataglance.asp.

p. 54 (margin): O'Higgins, *Madame*, 145.

p. 55: Charlotte Gere and Marina Vaizey, *Great Women Collectors* (London: Philip Wilson, 1999), 158.

p. 56 (margin): O'Higgins, *Madame*, 275.

p. 56 (first): "Helena Rubinstein Foundation: About Helena Rubinstein," http://fdncenter.org/grantmaker/rubinstein/about.html.

p. 56 (second): Lewis, *Miss Elizabeth Arden*, 306.

Chapter Three

p. 61: Lewis, *Miss Elizabeth Arden*, 35.

p. 64: Lewis, *Miss Elizabeth Arden*, 56.

p. 65 (margin): Lewis, *Miss Elizabeth Arden*, 252.

p. 65 (first): Lewis, *Miss Elizabeth Arden*, 58.

p. 65 (second): "Elizabeth Arden: Our Heritage," http://www.elizabetharden.com/heritage/early_start.asp.

p. 69: Lewis, *Miss Elizabeth Arden*, 136.

p. 71: Lewis, *Miss Elizabeth Arden*, 188.

p. 73: Lewis, *Miss Elizabeth Arden*, 278.

p. 74: Lewis, *Miss Elizabeth Arden*, 282.

Chapter Four

p. 85 (margin): Fred E. Basten, *Max Factor's Hollywood: Glamour, Movies, Make-up* (Santa Monica, Calif.: W. Quay Hays, 1995), 32.

p. 87: Basten, *Max Factor's Hollywood*, 150.

p. 88: "Maybelline: Early Successes," http://www.maybelline.com/us/success.html.

p. 93 (margin): Basten, *Max Factor's Hollywood*, 41.

Chapter Five

p. 95 (caption): Andrew Tobias, *Fire and Ice: The Story of Charles Revson—the Man Who Built the Revlon Empire* (New York: William Morrow, 1975), 126.

pp. 98-99: Tobias, *Fire and Ice*, 57.

p. 99 (margin): Tobias, *Fire and Ice*, 93.

p. 102: Tobias, *Fire and Ice*, 63.

p. 103 (margin): O'Higgins, *Madame*, 51.

p. 103 (first): Lee Israel, *Estée Lauder: Beyond the Magic* (New York: Macmillan, 1985), 63.

p. 103 (second): Tobias, *Fire and Ice*, 242.

p. 104 (margin): Lewis, *Miss Elizabeth Arden*, 257.

p. 107 (caption): Tobias, *Fire and Ice*, 130.

p. 110 (caption): Tobias, *Fire and Ice*, 86.

pp. 110-111: "Stahl Succeeds Nugent as Revlon President, CEO," http://www.chaindrugreview.com/articles/Stahl_succeeds_Nugent.html.

Chapter Six

p. 118 (margin): Estée Lauder, *Estée: A Success Story* (New York: Random House, 1985), 39.

p. 119: Lauder, *Estée*, 38.

p. 121: Lauder, *Estée,* 45.

p. 124: Lauder, *Estée,* 50.

Chapter Seven

p. 131 (caption): Anita Roddick, *Business as Unusual* (London: Thorsons, 2000), 101.

p. 132 (margin): Anita Roddick, *Body and Soul: Profits with Principles, the Amazing Success Story of Anita Roddick and The Body Shop* (New York: Crown, 1991), 43.

p. 139: Roddick, *Body and Soul*, 95.

p. 143: Roddick, *Body and Soul*, 149.

p. 144 (margin): Roddick, *Business as Unusual*, 70.

p. 144: Roddick, *Body and Soul*, 151.

p. 147 (margin): Roddick, *Body and Soul*, 10.

p. 147 (first): Roddick, *Business as Unusual*, 170.

p. 147 (second): Roddick, *Business as Unusual*, 172.

INDEX

ABOUT THE AUTHOR

Jacqueline C. Kent is a Jamaican-born author and freelance writer. She is the author of *Business Builders in Fashion*, also from The Oliver Press. She has a master's degree in Latin American history and gender studies and lives with her husband and two children in Reno, Nevada.

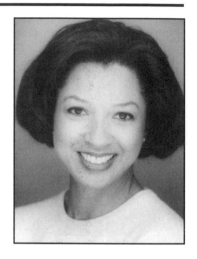

PHOTO CREDITS

Avon Products, Inc.: pp. 26, 37

The Body Shop International PLC: pp. 130 (Brian Moody), 133, 136, 137, 138, 141 (Sophia Evans), 142 (Clive Boursnell), 143 (Newscast), 146, back cover (both)

The Charles H. Revson Foundation: p. 94

Chicago Historical Society: p. 20

Corbis: p. 21 (Rick Maiman)

Elizabeth Arden Archives: pp. 2, 58, 64, 68, 70, 72, 73, 74

The Estée Lauder Companies, Inc.: pp. 112, 116, 119, 120, 122, 123, 125, 126, 129

Hagely Museum and Library: pp. 29, 31, 32, 33, 34

Helena Rubinstein Archives: cover, pp. 44, 49, 50, 55, 57

Helena Rubinstein Foundation: pp. 40, 46, 48, 51, 52

Library of Congress: pp. 6, 9, 10, 13, 16

Madame C. J. Walker Collection, Indiana Historical Society Library: pp. 17, 19 (both)

N. W. Ayer Advertising Agency Records, Archives Center, National Museum of American History, Smithsonian Institution: p. 23

Procter & Gamble Corporate Archives: pp. 76, 78, 79, 82, 84, 86, 89, 90, 91, 92

Timepix: p. 107

Andrew Tobias: pp. 99, 103, 105, 106, 110